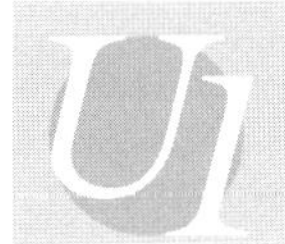

# UNIPAC One: *The Hospice/Palliative Medicine Approach to End-of-Life Care*

Second Edition

**Porter Storey, MD, FACP, FAAHPM**
Associate Professor of Medicine
Section of Geriatrics
Baylor College of Medicine

Consultant in the Department of Symptom Control and Palliative Care
University of Texas MD Anderson Cancer Center

Medical Director
Palliative Care Services
St. Luke's Episcopal Hospital
Houston, Texas

**Carol F. Knight, EdM**
Knight Consultants
Austin, Texas

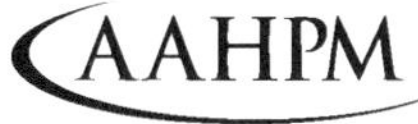


American Academy of Hospice and Palliative Medicine

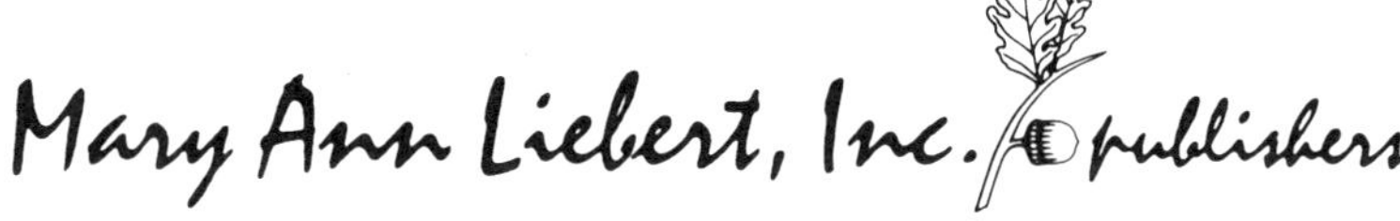

The information presented and opinions expressed herein are those of the authors and do not necessarily represent the views of the sponsor or its parent agencies, the National Institutes of Health, the United States Public Health Service, the reviewers, or a consensus of the members of the American Academy of Hospice and Palliative Medicine. Any recommendations made by the authors must be weighed against the physician's own clinical judgment, based on but not limited to such factors as the patient's condition, benefits versus risks of suggested treatment, and comparison with recommendations of pharmaceutical compendia and other authorities.



Published by Mary Ann Liebert, Inc. Publishers, 2 Madison Avenue, Larchmont, New York 10538-1962.



ISBN 0-913113-26-3

Printed in the United States of America

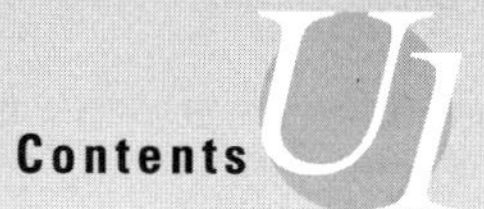

# Contents

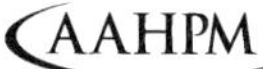

# Tables

# Figures

The authors and the American Academy of Hospice and Palliative Medicine (AAHPM) are deeply grateful to the following reviewers for their participation in the development of this component of the Academy's self-study curriculum, *Hospice/Palliative Care Training for Physicians: UNIPACs.* The reviewers' extensive comments and thoughtful suggestions greatly improved its contents. We want to express special gratitude to the following physicians who also recruited field testers and coordinated local testing of the UNIPAC: Gerald Holman, MD, Eli Perencevich, DO, and Julia Smith, MD. Finally, our special thanks to all the practicing physicians, fellows, residents, and medical students who participated in evaluating this component of the Academy's physician training curriculum.

**Samira K. Beckwith**
President
Hope Hospice
Ft. Myers, Florida

**Chris Cody, RNC, MSN**
Director of Professional and Regulatory Affairs
National Hospice Organization
Arlington, Virginia

**John W. Finn, MD**
Past President
Board of Directors, AAHPM
Medical Director
Hospice of Michigan
Southfield, Michigan

**Walter B. Forman, MD**
Past President
Board of Directors, AAHPM
Professor of Medicine and Geriatrics
University of New Mexico School of Medicine
Albuquerque, New Mexico

**Gerald H. Holman, MD**
Founding Chairman
Board of Trustees, AAHPM
Amarillo, Texas

**Eli N. Perencevich, DO**
Clinical Assistant Professor of Medicine
Ohio State University
Medical Director
Hospice of Columbus
Columbus, Ohio

**Julia L. Smith, MD**
Board of Directors, AAHPM
Division Chief, Oncology/Hematology
Genesee Hospital
Associate Professor, Oncology in Medicine
University of Rochester
Medical Director Hospice of Rochester
Rochester, New York

**David Wollner, MD**
Director, Palliative Care Services
VA New York Health Care System
Brooklyn, New York

# Academy's Physician Training Programs

The Academy recognizes the need for physician education on palliative medicine at the end of life and has designed its physician training programs to meet its own education goals, as well as those of the National Cancer Institute. The training programs include the following:

## Hospice/Palliative Medicine: Self-Study Program for Physicians

The Academy's self-study program consists of a series of monographs, or UNIPACs, each of which follows the recommended format for self-instructional learning, including behavioral objectives, a pretest, reading material, clinical situations for demonstrating knowledge application, a posttest, and references. The self-study program was made possible with federal funds from the National Cancer Institute's Cancer Education Grant Program, Grant CA66771. The following UNIPACs are approved for CME credit:

- *UNIPAC One: The Hospice/Palliative Medicine Approach to End-of-Life Care*
- *UNIPAC Two: Alleviating Psychological and Spiritual Pain in the Terminally Ill*
- *UNIPAC Three: Assessment and Treatment of Pain in the Terminally Ill*
- *UNIPAC Four: Management of Selected Non-pain Symptoms in the Terminally Ill*
- *UNIPAC Five: Caring for the Terminally Ill—Communication and the Physician's Role on the Interdisciplinary Team*
- *UNIPAC Six: Ethical and Legal Decision Making When Caring for the Terminally Ill*
- *UNIPAC Seven: The Hospice/Palliative Medicine Approach to Caring for Patients with AIDS*
- *UNIPAC Eight: The Hospice/Palliative Medicine Approach to Caring for Pediatric Patients*

Although the UNIPACs may be used when studying for the American Board of Hospice and Palliative Medicine's written examination for certification, they were not developed for that purpose. The Academy recommends that candidates for the examination review selected references listed at the end of each UNIPAC and other materials relevant to the examination.

### Pocket Guide to Hospice/Palliative Medicine

The *Pocket Guide to Hospice/Palliative Medicine* is a concise, clinically oriented reference for residents and practicing physicians. It consists primarily of tables and assessment tools from the Academy's self study program, *Hospice/Palliative Medicine: A Self-Study Program for Physicians.* Development of the Pocket Guide was made possible with federal funds from the National Cancer Institute's Cancer Education Grant Program, Grant CA66771.

### Hospice and Palliative Medicine: Core Curriculum and Review Syllabus

The Academy's core curriculum and review syllabus, *Hospice and Palliative Medicine: Core Curriculum and Review Syllabus,* presents the core elements of hospice and palliative medicine identified by the Institute of Medicine as essential for effective end-of-life care. The document consists of a series of modules, each of which includes a brief narrative summary of a specific topic, objectives, and references. The curriculum was the first one in the United States developed primarily by palliative medicine physicians.

### Primer of Palliative Care

The *Primer of Palliative Care* is a brief introduction to palliative care that covers the history of hospice, the basic elements of hospice and palliative care, pain and symptom management techniques, and alleviation of psychological, social, and spiritual distress. The Primer includes an annotated bibliography.

For more information on the Academy's physician training programs, call the AAHPM at (847) 375-4712 or fax (847) 375-6312.

## Continuing Medical Education

### Purpose

A UNIPAC is a packet of information formatted as a self-study program. It includes learning objectives, a pretest, reading material, clinical situations for demonstrating knowledge application, a posttest, and references. This self-study program is intended for physicians and physicians-in-training. It is designed to increase competence in palliative medical interventions for improving a patient's quality of life, particularly as death approaches. Specific, practical information is presented to help physicians assess and manage selected problems. After reading the UNIPAC, physicians are encouraged to seek additional training in hospice/palliative medicine.

## Learning Objectives

Upon completion of this continuing medical education program, a physician should be better able to:

- Define hospice/palliative medicine.
- Describe the roles of physicians practicing hospice/palliative medicine in hospice program settings.
- Educate patients, families, healthcare professionals, and the community about hospice/palliative medicine.
- Educate other physicians about effective palliative medicine interventions to control selected symptoms experienced by terminally ill patients in the home setting.
- Provide guidance when patients and families make decisions about end-of-life care.
- Help terminally ill patients and their families make treatment decisions congruent with their beliefs and values.
- Provide guidance when patients make the transition from curative to palliative care.
- Apply the National Hospice and Palliative Care Organization's (NHPCO's) Medical Guidelines for Determining Prognosis in Selected Non-Cancer Diseases when determining a patient's prognosis.
- Provide guidance when hospice/palliative care programs, patients, and families make decisions about eligibility for hospice care, discontinuation of hospice care, and the need for aggressive palliative treatments.
- Obtain allowable reimbursement when practicing hospice/palliative medicine.

## Recommended Procedure

To receive maximum benefit from this UNIPAC, the following procedure is recommended:

- Complete the pretest before reading the UNIPAC.
- Review the learning objectives.
- Study each section and the clinical situations.
- Review the correct responses to the pretest.
- Complete the posttest by marking your answers on the answer sheet.

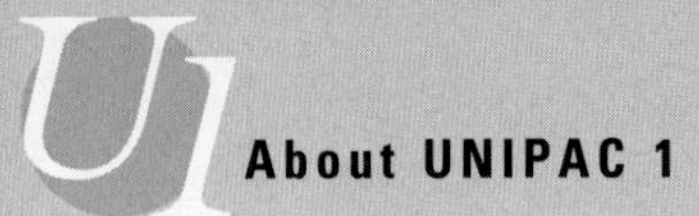


## Accreditation Statement

The American Academy of Hospice and Palliative Medicine (AAHPM) is accredited by the Accreditation Council for Continuing Medical Education (ACCME) to provide continuing medical education for physicians.

The AAHPM designates this continuing medical education activity for a maximum of six (6) hours in Category 1 towards the AMA Physician's Recognition Award.

Physicians are eligible to receive credit by completing and returning the evaluation form and the posttest answer sheet to the AAHPM. The Academy will keep a record of AMA/PRA Category 1 credit hours and the record will be provided on request; however, physicians are responsible for reporting their own Category 1 CME credits when applying for the AMA/PRA or for other certificates or credentials. Each physician should claim only those hours of credit that he or she actually spent in the activity.

## Disclosure

All faculty are required to disclose to program participants any relationship, including financial interest or affiliation(s), with a commercial company, as well as discussion of unlabeled uses. The program authors have disclosed information on sources of funding for research, consulting agreements, offices in professional associations, financial interests, and stock ownership.

**Porter Storey, MD,** once served on the speakers' bureau for Purdue Pharmaceuticals and has received research support from the National Cancer Institute. **Carol F. Knight, EdM,** has received research support from the National Cancer Institute.

## Review and Revision

Reviewed and re-approved by the American Academy of Hospice and Palliative Medicine's Publications and CME Committees: May 2002.

## Term of Offering

The release date for the second edition of this UNIPAC is February, 2003, and the expiration date is December 31, 2006. Final date to request credit is December 31, 2006.

## Posttest Pass Rate

The posttest pass rate is 75%.

## Additional Information

Additional information is available from the American Academy of Hospice and Palliative Medicine, where staff can direct you to physicians specializing in end-of-life care.

*This self-study program was supported in part by federal funds from the National Cancer Institute's Cancer Education Grant Program, Grant CA66771.*

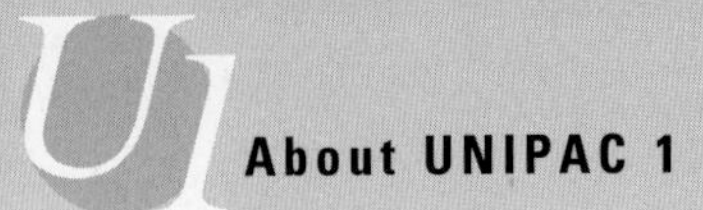


# Evaluation Form

Use this evaluation form to rate the UNIPAC that you have completed according to the five criteria listed and then mail or fax the form to the Academy at the address below. To receive CME credit, follow the same procedure.

| | | | | |
|---|---|---|---|---|
| Currency of information | __Excellent | __Good | __Fair | __Poor |
| Clarity of presentation | __Excellent | __Good | __Fair | __Poor |
| Content of material | __Excellent | __Good | __Fair | __Poor |
| Effectiveness of teaching method | __Excellent | __Good | __Fair | __Poor |
| Relevance to my practice | __Excellent | __Good | __Fair | __Poor |

Suggestions for improving the enduring material:

Mail or fax to:
American Academy of Hospice and Palliative Medicine
4700 W. Lake Avenue
Glenview, Illinois 60025-1485
Phone: 847/375-4761
Fax: 847/375-4777

# Pretest

Before proceeding, complete the following multiple-choice items. The correct responses are included at the end of the UNIPAC.

1. **All the following statements about the palliative model of care are true except which one?**
   A. A palliative intervention is indicated if it controls symptoms and relieves suffering.
   B. Emphasis is placed on knowing the patient's values, beliefs, and concerns.
   C. The primary goal is cure of the patient's disease.
   D. The subjective experiences of patients are valued as highly as objective data from laboratory tests.

2. **All the following definitions are true except which one?**
   A. Palliative care is the term used to describe whole-person care provided by an interdisciplinary team of healthcare professionals.
   B. Palliative treatments enhance comfort and improve a patient's quality of life.
   C. Therapies such as bone marrow transplantation or craniotomy for resection of metastases cannot be palliative interventions.
   D. Hospice programs provide palliative care to terminally ill patients 24 hours a day, 7 days a week in both home and facility-based settings.

3. **All the following are essential components of hospice/palliative medicine except which one?**
   A. Alleviating the suffering of patients and family members
   B. Helping patients and families make the transition from illness to death to bereavement
   C. Focusing solely on the physical aspects of suffering
   D. Participating in the patient's search for meaning and hope

4. **The principles of hospice care developed by Dr. Cicely Saunders include all the following except which one?**
   A. Research is inappropriate in hospice settings.
   B. A team of clinical professionals is needed to control symptoms.

C. Home care is a vital component of hospice care.

D. Teaching all aspects of terminal care is an essential component of a hospice physician's responsibilities.

**5. All the following statements about hospice/palliative care are true except which one?**

A. Each patient's beliefs, values, and concerns should be respected regardless of race, religion, sexual orientation, or financial status.

B. Hospice/palliative care interventions should be based on the results of careful research.

C. People, especially those who are suffering, rarely need help articulating their needs, values, concerns and fears.

D. Skillful interdisciplinary interventions can help to alleviate suffering.

**6. The NHPCO Standards of Care for Hospice Programs include all the following except which one?**

A. The hospice interdisciplinary team collaborates continuously with the patient's attending physician.

B. Hospice programs can offer fewer services to patients residing in nursing facilities.

C. Hospice programs offer palliative care services to terminally ill patients regardless of their diagnosis, availability of a primary caregiver, or ability to pay.

D. Hospice care services are available 24 hours a day, 7 days a week.

**7. All the following statements about the responsibilities of physicians practicing hospice/palliative medicine are true except which one?**

A. Provide guidance and support as patients make the transition from curative to palliative care.

B. Provide information about diagnosis, prognosis, and treatment options.

C. Give selflessly to patients and their family members, staff, and team members.

D. Participate in team meetings.

**8. The rules for making prudent judgments include all the following except which one?**

A. Physicians should refrain from offering an opinion about a treatment because they may influence a patient's choice.

B. Physicians should pay increased attention to patient vulnerability.

C. Physicians should maintain a healthy respect for moral ambiguity.

D. Physicians should encourage patient autonomy.

**9. All the following statements about Dr. Cicely Saunders are true except which one?**

A. Dr. Saunders is usually credited with developing the art and science of modern hospice care.

B. Dr. Saunders founded the world-renowned St. Christopher's Hospice in England.

C. Dr. Saunders developed the concept of total pain, which describes the all-encompassing physical, emotional, spiritual, and social pain experienced by many dying patients.

D. Dr. Saunders was more concerned with general concepts than with the details of patient care or research.

**10. All the following statements about Dr. Elizabeth Kübler-Ross are true except which one?**

A. Her book, *On Death and Dying,* was a best-seller and sparked widespread interest in the care of dying patients.

B. She described the conspiracy of silence that surrounds dying people.

C. She believed that patients always experience five stages of dying in exactly the same order: denial, anger, bargaining, depression, and acceptance.

D. She interviewed dying patients about their reactions to dying.

**11. All the following are barriers to effective end-of-life care except which one?**

A. Misconceptions about opioids on the part of many healthcare professionals, e.g., opioids cause addiction

B. Lack of effective medications to control pain

C. Lack of medical school emphasis on end-of-life care

D. The widespread belief among physicians that there is nothing they can do when patients are terminally ill

**12. In the United States, all the following are barriers to palliative care for terminally ill patients in the home setting except which one?**

A. Lack of adequate insurance coverage

B. Inadequate numbers of hospice programs in most cities

C. Lack of physician skill in pain management and communication

D. Lack of coordination of services for nonhospice patients

**13. All the following statements about managing symptoms of advanced cancer in patients in the home setting are true except which one?**

A. When insomnia is a problem for a confused patient, major tranquilizers such as thioridazine (Mellaril) or chlorpromazine (Thorazine) may be more useful than benzodiazepine hypnotics.

B. When convulsions or acute delusional states are a problem, most families can learn to use subcutaneous routes to deliver medications such as phenobarbital or haloperidol.

C. When fecal incontinence is a problem, use osmotic laxatives like lactulose and sorbitol.

D. When bleeding is a problem, avoid NSAIDs and Coumadin, and control hypertension aggressively.

**14. All the following statements about ethical issues in the home setting are true except which one?**

A. Patients have a right to know their diagnosis, prognosis, and treatment options.

B. Physicians can share confidential patient information with other members of the interdisciplinary team without the patient's consent.

C. Treating the patient's symptoms just to relieve family distress can be an ethically correct choice in some situations.

D. Patients should not be sedated against their will.

**15. All the following statements about the costs of hospice care are true except which one?**

A. Definitive studies have proved that hospice care reduces healthcare costs throughout the illness trajectory.

B. Hospice care and the use of advance directives may save 25% to 40% of healthcare costs during the last month of a patient's life.

C. Because comprehensive hospice/palliative care involves complex, interdisciplinary interventions, it may not be less expensive than conventional care throughout the illness trajectory.

D. Aggressive palliative interventions may require large quantities of expensive medications, radiation therapy, or surgical interventions.

**16. All the following statements about the Medicare Hospice Benefit are true except which one?**

A. To receive the Medicaid Hospice Benefit for coverage of a terminal illness, patients waive traditional Medicare hospital coverage for the terminal illness.

B. The Medicare Hospice Benefit pays hospice programs at a per diem rate to cover all healthcare costs related to the terminal diagnosis, including prescription medications.

C. After choosing the Medicare Hospice Benefit, patients are still covered by traditional Medicare Part A for problems unrelated to the terminal diagnosis.

D. More than 80% of elderly patients have chosen the comprehensive coverage offered by the Medicare Hospice Benefit.

**17. All the following statements about patient eligibility for the Medicare Hospice Benefit are true except which one?**

A. In most cases, the patient must be 65 years of age or older and be eligible for Medicare Part A.

B. The patient must have a primary caregiver in the home.

C. In most cases, the patient must be certified as terminally ill by two physicians.

D. Care related to the patient's terminal illness must be provided by a Medicare-certified hospice program.

**18. All the following statements about the Medicare Hospice Benefit are true except which one?**

A. The revised benefit consists of two 90-day periods followed by an unlimited number of 60-day periods.

B. Patients may revoke the hospice benefit at any time, but revocation results in the loss of all remaining days in that benefit period.

C. When patients revoke the hospice benefit, traditional Medicare Part A is immediately available to them.

D. At the end of each benefit period, patients are automatically eligible for continuation of the hospice benefit.

**19. All the following statements about the Medicare Hospice Benefit are true except which one?**

A. The benefit pays a per diem that covers all medicines, biologicals, durable medical equipment, and medical supplies needed to palliate symptoms related to the terminal illness.

B. The benefit includes coverage for services from home health aide and homemakers.

C. The benefit covers the cost of a patient's room and board in a nursing home.

D. The benefit covers respite stays for patients to relieve family member distress.

**20. All the following statements about the Medicare Hospice Benefit are true except which one?**

A. The benefit provides per diem reimbursement based on four levels of care: routine home care, continuous home care, general inpatient care, and respite care.

B. Continuous home care is for crisis management of acute symptoms so patients can remain at home; at least 51% of the care must require the services of licensed nurses.

C. The per diem rate for routine home care is paid regardless of the number of services provided on a particular day.

D. Medicare sets no limits on reimbursement for needed services.

**21. All following statements about Medicare Hospice Benefit reimbursement for physician services are true except which one?**

A. Administrative services provided by physicians employed by the hospice are not included in the hospice program's per diem rate and can be billed separately.

B. Physicians who are hospice employees or who provide direct patient care services under arrangement with the hospice bill the hospice program directly for professional services and are reimbursed at an agreed-upon rate.

C. Attending physicians who are not hospice employees but provide direct patient care services bill Medicare Part B for professional services, just as they would for nonhospice patients.

D. Consulting physicians who provide patient care services bill the hospice program directly for professional services and are reimbursed by the program at an agreed-upon rate.

**22. All the following statements about Medicare Hospice Benefit reimbursement for physicians are true except which one?**

A. An attending physician bills Medicare Part B for professional services related to chemotherapy or radiation therapy.

B. A consultant physician bills the hospice program directly for professional services related to chemotherapy or radiation therapy.

C. The attending physician bills Medicare Part A for the cost of chemotherapy drugs.

D. When consulting physicians bill the hospice program for professional services, the program is reimbursed by Medicare Part A for 100% of the Medicare allowable amount.

**23. All the following statements about ethical issues related to hospice/palliative care are true except which one?**

A. Increasing religious and cultural diversity requires careful attention to the values, needs, and concerns of each patient.

B. When news of a life-threatening illness affects a patient's ability to make decisions, the physician should help the patient articulate his or her beliefs, values, and goals.

C. Physicians are obligated to honestly and compassionately tell patients as much as they want to know about their diagnosis and prognosis.

D. Patients are obliged to participate in research projects that may improve hospice/palliative care for others.

**24. All the following statements about hospice program policies are true except which one?**

A. It is permissible to deny hospice services to terminally ill patients who threaten the personal safety of hospice staff.

B. Hospice programs can ethically discharge patients whose symptoms are too expensive to manage.

C. Medicare-certified hospice programs must provide all covered services included in the patient's Plan of Care that are reasonable and necessary for the palliation and management of a terminal illness.

D. To improve access for underserved populations, hospice program policies should train staff to communicate effectively with patients from various ethnic groups and religious traditions.

*In most cases, dying, like birthing, is a process requiring assistance. It is an event that asks us to be present for one another with heart and mind, bringing not only practical help as necessary, but also attentive awareness and appreciation of the individual involved. At its finest, it elicits from us the frankly and fully offered human companionship that brings positive benefits, and a kind of joy, to any shared venture.*

— Sandol Stoddard[1]

*We are a culture that denies death . . . therefore we are all walking towards death backwards! It is better to turn around.*

—Michael Meade[2]

# Curative versus Palliative Models of Care

As palliative medicine emerges as a field of specialization,[3] its role and goals must be more clearly understood. The goals of medicine are varied; they include relief of suffering, health promotion, and injury prevention.[4] In medical education, one goal— the cure of disease— receives more attention than any other but no widely accepted definition of the *curative model* of medical care exists.[5] Essentially, it is an approach to clinical medicine that focuses narrowly on eradicating an illness or disease. As Fox states, "In its purest form, the curative model concentrates solely on the goal of cure and in the process neglects medicine's other goals."[6, p.761]

Medicine's limited focus on treating disease was established during the Renaissance, when religious concerns threatened scientific progress. The Cartesian separation of mind and body provided a solution to a religious–scientific impasse by allocating the patient's body to science and the patient's mind to the church. However, the expedient separation of body from mind resulted in the long-standing medical illusion that treating a disease can be separated from caring for the person who is suffering.[7] The unfortunate long-term results of medicine's narrowed focus include:

- Deconstruction of suffering (only physical pain is real)
- Devaluation of important components of the patient's personhood (only the body is real)
- Overreliance on seemingly objective data from diagnostic procedures such as electrocardiograms or x-rays (only objective measurable data are real and trustworthy, not the patient's description of symptoms)

- Loss of empathetic communication skills (only the patient's body is real and of interest, so there is little need to communicate with the person experiencing the illness)

Despite apparent acceptance of the need for whole-person care and greater appreciation of the mind–body connections that make up personhood, the separation of mind and body continues to pervade medical practice and clinical training.[8] However, changing societal expectations are contributing to a reevaluation of medicine's role. Instead of defining physicians solely as technological miracle workers, both clinicians and society are beginning to view the physician's role as one that includes both treating illness ***and*** caring for the person who is experiencing the illness.

The palliative model of care recognizes the importance not only of cure, but also of symptom control and relief of suffering. Table 1 compares the characteristics of curative and palliative care. For information on incorporating palliative care into the healthcare system, see the section "Models for Integrating Hospice/Palliative Care into the Healthcare System" on page 37.

**Table 1: Characteristics of Curative and Palliative Care Models[6]**

| Curative Model | Palliative Model |
|---|---|
| The primary goal is cure. | The primary goal is relief of suffering. |
| The object of analysis is the disease process. | The object of analysis is the patient and the family. |
| Symptoms are treated primarily as clues to diagnosis. | Distressing symptoms are treated as entities in themselves. |
| Primary value is placed on measurable data, e.g., laboratory tests. | Both measurable and subjective data are valued. |
| Tends to devalue information that is subjective, immeasurable, or unverifiable. | Values the patient's experience of an illness. |
| Therapy is medically indicated if it eradicates or slows the progression of disease. | Therapy is medically indicated if it controls symptoms and relieves suffering. |
| The patient's body is differentiated from the mind. | The patient is viewed as a complex being consisting of physical, emotional, social, and spiritual dimensions. |
| Patients are viewed as collections of parts, so there is little need to get to know the whole person. | Treatment is congruent with the values, beliefs, and concerns of the patient and family. |
| Death is the ultimate failure. | Enabling a patient to live fully and comfortably until he or she dies is a success. |

# Definitions of Words Associated with Hospice/Palliative Care

To help to establish a common ground of meaning, UNIPAC One begins with definitions of several words associated with hospice/palliative medicine; see Table 2.

## Summary of Key Points

- The term *palliative care* refers to whole-person care for patients whose diseases are not responsive to curative treatment. Palliative care may be provided by an interdisciplinary team of physicians, nurses, social workers, chaplains, and other healthcare professionals
- The term *palliative medicine* refers to a medical specialty that focuses on patients whose diseases are not responsive to curative treatment. In the United States, physicians practicing palliative medicine in hospice settings often refer to their area of expertise as *hospice/palliative medicine.*
- *Palliative medicine* includes very aggressive measures to control pain and other distressing symptoms.
- The term *hospice* refers to a program that provides coordinated comprehensive palliative care for terminally ill patients and their families, whether in home or facility settings, through an interdisciplinary team of healthcare professionals.

The term *supportive care* is used in several healthcare settings, but its meaning varies. Some healthcare professionals use the term supportive care when referring to comprehensive interventions designed to alleviate a patient's physical, psychological, social, and spiritual distress. Oncologists more often use the term when referring to medical interventions that may alleviate or prevent tumor-induced symptoms, e.g., the use of hematopoietic growth factors, granulocyte transfusions, autologous bone marrow transplants, and chemotherapy agents.

More recently, the term palliative chemotherapy has been used to describe chemotherapy treatments designed to relieve cancer-induced symptoms. To avoid confusion, the term supportive care is not used in this UNIPAC. Instead, the terms *hospice care* or *hospice/palliative care* are used interchangeably when referring to comprehensive care for terminally ill patients.

**Table 2: Definitions Associated with Hospice/Palliative Care**

- **Palliative care** is active total care of patients whose diseases are not responsive to curative treatment. Symptom control is paramount and includes the alleviation of symptoms, whether they are physical, psychological, social, or spiritual. Total palliative care usually involves an interdisciplinary team of healthcare professionals who provide coordinated medical, nursing, social work, and spiritual care services. The goal of palliative care is to achieve the best possible quality of life for patients and their families. Many aspects of palliative care are also applicable earlier in the course of an illness in conjunction with anticancer treatment.[9]
- **Palliative medicine** is the study and management of patients with active, progressive, far-advanced disease for whom the prognosis is limited and the focus of care is the quality of life.[10]
- **Hospice/palliative medicine** is the study and management of patients with active, progressive, far-advanced disease for whom the prognosis is limited and the focus of care is quality of life. The discipline recognizes the multidimensional nature of suffering, responds with care that addresses all dimensions of suffering, and communicates in language that conveys mutuality, respect, and interdependence[11] (adapted from the American Board of Hospice and Palliative Medicine).
- **Palliative treatments** are treatments and interventions that enhance comfort and improve the quality of a patient's life. No specific therapy is excluded from consideration. The test of a palliative treatment lies in the agreement by the patient, physician, primary caregiver, and an interdisciplinary team of healthcare professionals that the treatment's expected outcome is relief from distressing symptoms, easing of pain, and enhancement of quality of life. The decision to intervene with an active palliative treatment is based on the treatment's ability to meet the stated goals rather than its effect on the underlying disease. The needs of each patient are continually assessed, and all treatment options are explored and evaluated within the context of the patient's values and symptoms[12] (adapted from the National Hospice and Palliative Care Organization, NHPCO, formerly the National Hospice Organization).
- **Hospice programs** provide palliative care to terminally ill patients and supportive services to their families and significant others, 24 hours a day, 7 days a week, in both home and facility-based settings. Physical, social, spiritual, and emotional care is provided during the last stages of illness, during the dying process, and during bereavement by a medically directed interdisciplinary team consisting of patients and families, professionals, and volunteers[12] (adapted from the NHPCO).

## Philosophy of Hospice/Palliative Care

*. . . [T]he alleviation of suffering is the warrant of medicine and its test of adequacy . . . it is a test that contemporary medicine fails despite the brilliance of its science and its awesome technological power.*

—Eric J. Cassel[13]

*The hospice philosophy of care affirms support and care for people in the last phases of incurable disease so that they may live as fully and as comfortably as possible. Hospice recognizes dying as part of the normal process of living and focuses on maintaining the quality of remaining life. Hospice affirms life and neither hastens nor postpones death. Hospice exists in the hope and belief that through appropriate care, and the promotion of a caring community sensitive to their needs, patients and their families may be free to attain a degree of mental and spiritual preparation for death that is satisfactory to them.*

—NHO[12]

Evidence indicates that the moment of death often is a welcome relief, but the process of dying can be hard work. Like women giving birth, people who are dying usually require practical assistance and caring presence.[1] Some people associate hospice/palliative care programs only with death care, but this view is mistaken. Instead, programs focus on improving quality of life and helping patients live life to the fullest until death occurs. The ultimate goal of hospice/palliative care is to alleviate suffering and provide "safe passage" as patients make the transition from this life to whatever follows death.[14]

Palliative interventions are designed to provide comfort, not to cure disease or extend life. Because palliative interventions control distressing symptoms and provide psychological and spiritual support, they may prolong a patient's life while improving its quality. The essential components of hospice/palliative care include the following:

- Alleviating the suffering of patients and families by focusing on all aspects of total pain: physical, emotional, spiritual, and social pain
- Improving the patient's quality of life
- Helping patients and families to make the transition from health to illness to death to bereavement
- Participating in the patient's and family's search for meaning and hope
- Helping patients to achieve the developmental goals of the dying according to their specific needs and wishes

## Saunders's Principles of Hospice Care

Early in her career, Dr. Cicely Saunders, the founder of modern hospice care, developed the principles of hospice care listed in Table 3.[15] Dr. Saunders's principles suggest that hospice program policies should reflect the following values:

- Patients, family members, and healthcare professionals are more than collections of cells, bones, and blood; each is unique and has important physical, emotional, social, and spiritual needs.
- Each person's beliefs, values, and concerns should be respected regardless of nationality, race, religion, sexual orientation, disability, or financial status.
- Suffering people usually need help from caring, skilled professionals to articulate their needs, values, concerns, and fears.
- Suffering people benefit from skilled interdisciplinary interventions that alleviate physical, emotional, spiritual, and social pain.
- Palliative interventions should be based on the results of careful research.
- Continued professional and personal growth is important for all concerned.

**Table 3: Saunders's Principles of Hospice Care[15]**

- A clinical team is needed if expert control of symptoms is to be maintained.
- The hospice team involves the paramedical disciplines.
- Skilled and experienced team nursing is required.
- Methodical recording and analysis should monitor clinical practice and, with relevant research where possible, lead to soundly based practice and teaching.
- Some form of home care must be developed and fully integrated with the community services already established.
- A bereavement follow-up service should be included.
- Teaching in all aspects of terminal care should be included.
- Imaginative use of available architecture should create a supportive environment.
- An efficient and approachable administration is essential to any field of human need; it provides a sense of security to patients, families, and staff.
- Hospices should consider a mixed group of patients, including those with long-term progressive illnesses, chronic pain, and in some cases, frailty and old age.
- Readiness for the personal cost of commitment to a continuous search for meaning is essential.

# Quality of Life

## Assessing Quality of Life

Improving a patient's quality of life (QOL) is the ultimate goal of palliative medicine. Although a one-time score on an assessment scale does not provide reliable information about a patient's quality of life, comparing a patient's responses over time to the same assessment tool is likely to reveal important information. As patients cope with the effects of profound illness, their assessment scores are likely to diminish. However, significant decreases are less likely to occur when pain and other symptoms are effectively controlled, and when emotional and spiritual support are provided.

QOL assessments offer diagnostic and therapeutic benefits. In terms of diagnosis, assessments may reveal uncontrolled pain, the most reliable predictor of poor QOL. In terms of therapy, just the process of completing a QOL assessment tool can change a patient's perspective on issues related to living and dying, particularly as life comes to a close. In addition to tracking an individual's QOL over time, assessment tools are useful for comparing the QOL of large populations; for example, comparing the QOL of a large group of nursing home patients with that of a large group of patients in hospice/palliative care inpatient units. (See Tables 4 and 5 for examples of QOL scales.)

**Table 4: McGill Quality of Life Questionnaire[16]**

*Over the past two days,*

1. One troublesome symptom is ______________

| | | | | | | | | | | | | | |
|---|---|---|---|---|---|---|---|---|---|---|---|---|---|
| No problem | 0 | 1 | 2 | 3 | 4 | 5 | 6 | 7 | 8 | 9 | 10 | Tremendous problem |

2. Another troublesome symptom is ______________

| | | | | | | | | | | | | |
|---|---|---|---|---|---|---|---|---|---|---|---|---|
| No problem | 0 | 1 | 2 | 3 | 4 | 5 | 6 | 7 | 8 | 9 | 10 | Tremendous problem |

3. A third troublesome symptom is ______________

| | | | | | | | | | | | | |
|---|---|---|---|---|---|---|---|---|---|---|---|---|
| No problem | 0 | 1 | 2 | 3 | 4 | 5 | 6 | 7 | 8 | 9 | 10 | Tremendous problem |

4. Physically, I felt

| | | | | | | | | | | | | |
|---|---|---|---|---|---|---|---|---|---|---|---|---|
| Terrible | 0 | 1 | 2 | 3 | 4 | 5 | 6 | 7 | 8 | 9 | 10 | Well |

5. I was depressed

| | | | | | | | | | | | | |
|---|---|---|---|---|---|---|---|---|---|---|---|---|
| Not at all | 0 | 1 | 2 | 3 | 4 | 5 | 6 | 7 | 8 | 9 | 10 | Extremely |

6. I was nervous or worried

| | | | | | | | | | | | | |
|---|---|---|---|---|---|---|---|---|---|---|---|---|
| Not at all | 0 | 1 | 2 | 3 | 4 | 5 | 6 | 7 | 8 | 9 | 10 | Extremely |

7. How much of the time did you feel sad?

| | | | | | | | | | | | | |
|---|---|---|---|---|---|---|---|---|---|---|---|---|
| Never | 0 | 1 | 2 | 3 | 4 | 5 | 6 | 7 | 8 | 9 | 10 | Always |

8. When I think about the future, I am

| | | | | | | | | | | | | |
|---|---|---|---|---|---|---|---|---|---|---|---|---|
| Not afraid | 0 | 1 | 2 | 3 | 4 | 5 | 6 | 7 | 8 | 9 | 10 | Constantly terrified |

(*Continued*)

| | | | |
|---|---|---|---|
| 9. My personal existence is | | | |
| | Utterly meaningless and without purpose | 0 1 2 3 4 5 6 7 8 9 10 | Very purposeful and meaningful |
| 10. In achieving life goals, I have | | | |
| | Made no progress whatsoever | 0 1 2 3 4 5 6 7 8 9 10 | Progressed to complete fulfillment |
| 11. My life to this point has been | | | |
| | Completely worthless | 0 1 2 3 4 5 6 7 8 9 10 | Very worthwhile |
| 12. I have | | | |
| | No control over my life | 0 1 2 3 4 5 6 7 8 9 10 | Complete control over my life |
| 13. I feel good about myself as a person | | | |
| | Completely disagree | 0 1 2 3 4 5 6 7 8 9 10 | Completely agree |
| 14. To me, every day seems to be | | | |
| | A burden | 0 1 2 3 4 5 6 7 8 9 10 | A gift |
| 15. The world is | | | |
| | An impersonal, unfeeling place | 0 1 2 3 4 5 6 7 8 9 10 | Caring and responsive to my needs |
| 16. I feel supported | | | |
| | Not at all | 0 1 2 3 4 5 6 7 8 9 10 | Completely |

Cohen SR, Mount BM, Strobel MG, Bui F. The McGill Quality of Life Questionnaire; a measure of quality of life appropriate for people with advanced disease. A preliminary study of validity and acceptability. Palliat Med. 1995;9(3):207–219.

## Table 5: Measuring the Quality of Life of Seriously Ill Patients[17]

*Instructions to patient:*
I'd like you to think back over the last month. Please tell me the three physical symptoms or problems that have bothered you the most during that time. Some examples are pain, nausea, lack of energy, confusion, depression, anxiety, and shortness of breath.

Symptom #1__________________________

Symptom #3__________________________

Symptom #2__________________________

- If no symptoms were elicited, then state the following: "So, just to be sure, over the last month, you have had no physical or emotional symptoms that bothered you."
- If correct, skip to question #5.

Which of these symptoms or problems has bothered you the most this past week?

1. During the last week, how often have you experienced __________________?

| *Rarely* | *A few times* | *Fairly often* | *Very often* | *Most of the time* |
|---|---|---|---|---|
| 1 | 2 | 3 | 4 | 5 |

2. During the last week, on average, how severe has __________________ been?

| *Very mild* | *Mild* | *Moderate* | *Severe* | *Very severe* |
|---|---|---|---|---|
| 1 | 2 | 3 | 4 | 5 |

3. During the last week, how much has ________________ interfered with your ability to enjoy your life?

| *Not at all* | *A little bit* | *A moderate amount* | *Quite a bit* | *Completely* |
|---|---|---|---|---|
| 1 | 2 | 3 | 4 | 5 |

4. How worried are you about ________________ occurring in the future?

| *Not at all* | *A little bit* | *A moderate amount* | *Quite a bit* | *Completely* |
|---|---|---|---|---|
| 1 | 2 | 3 | 4 | 5 |

5. In general, how important are your PHYSICAL SYMPTOMS OR PROBLEMS to your overall quality of life?

| *Not at all* | *A little bit* | *A moderate amount* | *Quite a bit* | *Completely* |
|---|---|---|---|---|
| 1 | 2 | 3 | 4 | 5 |

**Below is a list of statements that other people with a serious illness have said may be important. Please tell me how true each statement is for you.**

6. I have as much information as I want about my illness.

| *Not at all* | *A little bit* | *A moderate amount* | *Quite a bit* | *Completely* |
|---|---|---|---|---|
| 1 | 2 | 3 | 4 | 5 |

7. Although I cannot control certain aspects of my illness, I have a sense of control about my treatment decisions.

| *Not at all* | *A little bit* | *A moderate amount* | *Quite a bit* | *Completely* |
|---|---|---|---|---|
| 1 | 2 | 3 | 4 | 5 |

8. I participate as much as I want in the decisions about my care.

| *Not at all* | *A little bit* | *A moderate amount* | *Quite a bit* | *Completely* |
|---|---|---|---|---|
| 1 | 2 | 3 | 4 | 5 |

9. Beyond my illness, my doctor has a sense of who I am as a person.

| *Not at all* | *A little bit* | *A moderate amount* | *Quite a bit* | *Completely* |
|---|---|---|---|---|
| 1 | 2 | 3 | 4 | 5 |

10. In general, I know what to expect about the course of my illness.

| *Not at all* | *A little bit* | *A moderate amount* | *Quite a bit* | *Completely* |
|---|---|---|---|---|
| 1 | 2 | 3 | 4 | 5 |

11. As my illness progresses, I know where to go to get answers to my questions.

| *Not at all* | *A little bit* | *A moderate amount* | *Quite a bit* | *Completely* |
|---|---|---|---|---|
| 1 | 2 | 3 | 4 | 5 |

12. In general, how important is feeling like an ACTIVE PARTICIPANT in your HEALTH CARE to your overall quality of life?

| *Not at all* | *A little bit* | *A moderate amount* | *Quite a bit* | *Completely* |
|---|---|---|---|---|
| 1 | 2 | 3 | 4 | 5 |

13. I spend as much time as I want with my family.

| *Not at all* | *A little bit* | *A moderate amount* | *Quite a bit* | *Completely* |
|---|---|---|---|---|
| 1 | 2 | 3 | 4 | 5 |

14. There is someone in my life with whom I can share my deepest thoughts.

| *Not at all* | *A little bit* | *A moderate amount* | *Quite a bit* | *Completely* |
|---|---|---|---|---|
| 1 | 2 | 3 | 4 | 5 |

15. In general, how important are your PERSONAL RELATIONSHIPS to your overall quality of life?

| *Not at all* | *A little bit* | *A moderate amount* | *Quite a bit* | *Completely* |
|---|---|---|---|---|
| 1 | 2 | 3 | 4 | 5 |

16. In general, how important is feeling CONNECTED TO OTHERS to your overall quality of life?

| *Not at all* | *A little bit* | *A moderate amount* | *Quite a bit* | *Completely* |
|---|---|---|---|---|
| 1 | 2 | 3 | 4 | 5 |

17. Thoughts of dying frighten me.

| *Not at all* | *A little bit* | *A moderate amount* | *Quite a bit* | *Completely* |
|---|---|---|---|---|
| 1 | 2 | 3 | 4 | 5 |

*(Continued)*

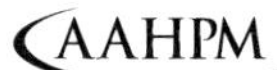

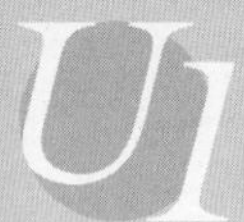


18. I worry that my family is not prepared to cope with the future.

| *Not at all* | *A little bit* | *A moderate amount* | *Quite a bit* | *Completely* |
|---|---|---|---|---|
| 1 | 2 | 3 | 4 | 5 |

19. I have regrets about the way I have lived my life.

| *Not at all* | *A little bit* | *A moderate amount* | *Quite a bit* | *Completely* |
|---|---|---|---|---|
| 1 | 2 | 3 | 4 | 5 |

20 At times, I worry that I *will be* a burden to my family.

| *Not at all* | *A little bit* | *A moderate amount* | *Quite a bit* | *Completely* |
|---|---|---|---|---|
| 1 | 2 | 3 | 4 | 5 |

21. I worry about the financial strain caused by my illness.

| *Not at all* | *A little bit* | *A moderate amount* | *Quite a bit* | *Completely* |
|---|---|---|---|---|
| 1 | 2 | 3 | 4 | 5 |

22. In general, how important are CONCERNS ABOUT THE FUTURE to your overall quality of life?

| *Not at all* | *A little bit* | *A moderate amount* | *Quite a bit* | *Completely* |
|---|---|---|---|---|
| 1 | 2 | 3 | 4 | 5 |

23. I have been able to say important things to those close to me.

| *Not at all* | *A little bit* | *A moderate amount* | *Quite a bit* | *Completely* |
|---|---|---|---|---|
| 1 | 2 | 3 | 4 | 5 |

24. I make a positive difference in the lives of others.

| *Not at all* | *A little bit* | *A moderate amount* | *Quite a bit* | *Completely* |
|---|---|---|---|---|
| 1 | 2 | 3 | 4 | 5 |

25. I have been able to help others through time together, gifts, or wisdom.

| *Not at all* | *A little bit* | *A moderate amount* | *Quite a bit* | *Completely* |
|---|---|---|---|---|
| 1 | 2 | 3 | 4 | 5 |

26. I have been able to share important things with my family.

| *Not at all* | *A little bit* | *A moderate amount* | *Quite a bit* | *Completely* |
|---|---|---|---|---|
| 1 | 2 | 3 | 4 | 5 |

27. Despite my illness, I have a sense of meaning in my life.

| *Not at all* | *A little bit* | *A moderate amount* | *Quite a bit* | *Completely* |
|---|---|---|---|---|
| 1 | 2 | 3 | 4 | 5 |

28. I feel at peace.

| *Not at all* | *A little bit* | *A moderate amount* | *Quite a bit* | *Completely* |
|---|---|---|---|---|
| 1 | 2 | 3 | 4 | 5 |

29. In general, how important is CONTRIBUTING TO OTHERS to your overall quality of life?

| *Not at all* | *A little bit* | *A moderate amount* | *Quite a bit* | *Completely* |
|---|---|---|---|---|
| 1 | 2 | 3 | 4 | 5 |

30. In general, how important is the feeling that your LIFE IS COMPLETE to your overall quality of life?

| *Not at all* | *A little bit* | *A moderate amount* | *Quite a bit* | *Completely* |
|---|---|---|---|---|
| 1 | 2 | 3 | 4 | 5 |

Now, I have one last question.

31. How would you rate your OVERALL QUALITY OF LIFE?

| *Very Poor* | *Poor* | *Fair* | *Good* | *Excellent* |
|---|---|---|---|---|
| 1 | 2 | 3 | 4 | 5 |

Tulsky JA, Steinhauser KE, Bosworth HB, Clipp EC, McNeilly M, Christakis NA. Assessment of a new instrument to measure quality of life at the end of life. J Pall Med. 2002;5(1):206. Abstract. Reprinted with permission from Tulsky JA, et al.

# NHPCO Principles of Hospice Care

To ensure the provision of quality hospice/palliative care, the National Hospice and Palliative Care Organization (NHPCO), formerly the National Hospice Organization (NHO), developed principles and standards of care.[12,16] Table 6 lists the NHPCO's principles of care and selected operational guidelines.

**Table 6: NHPCO Principles of Care and Selected Operational Guidelines[11,15]**

- **Hospice programs offer palliative care to all terminally ill people and their families** regardless of age, gender, nationality, race, creed, sexual orientation, disability, diagnosis, availability of a primary caregiver, or ability to pay. *Guidelines:* Admission policies should not exclude potentially high-cost patients, discriminate against any needed palliative therapy or treatment, or exclude patients based on the safety of their neighborhoods, modality of therapy, psychiatric symptoms, payor source, ability to pay an allowable co-pay, or presence of supplemental insurance.
- **The unit of care in hospice is the patient and family.** Guidelines: Patients should not be excluded from care due to the presence of difficult family members.
- **A highly qualified, specially trained team of hospice professionals and volunteers work together** to meet the physiological, psychological, social, spiritual, and economic needs of hospice patients and families facing terminal illness and bereavement. *Guidelines:* Programs should develop caseload policies that ensure the provision of high-quality care. See "Reduce Organizational Barriers to Quality Hospice Care" on page 92.
- **The hospice interdisciplinary team collaborates continuously with the patient's attending physician** to develop and maintain a patient-directed, individualized plan of care. Medical interventions proposed to alleviate symptoms of a terminal illness should be evaluated by the attending physician, hospice medical director, team, patient, and family.to determine the likely impact on the patient's quality of life, the value of the treatment to the patient, and its congruence with the goals of palliative care.
- **Hospice provides a safe, coordinated program of palliative and supportive care** in a variety of settings from the time of admission through bereavement, with a focus on keeping terminally ill patients in their own homes for as long as possible. *Guidelines:* Programs should provide home health aide, homemaker, and volunteer services adequate to meet the patient's needs.
- **Hospice care is available 24 hours a day, 7 days a week**. Services continue without interruption when the patient's care setting changes. *Guidelines:* Patients should be evaluated and, if appropriate, admitted within one working day of the patient's or family's request for hospice services. Hospice programs should be able to admit patients 7 days a week and should demonstrate appropriate patient access to all levels of care. Programs should follow suggested criteria when discharging a patient and should not request that patients revoke the hospice benefit due to hospitalization.

(*Continued*)

- **Hospice is accountable for the appropriate allocation and utilization of its resources** to provide optimal care consistent with patient and family needs. *Guidelines:* The same level, intensity, and mix of services should be provided to patients whether they reside in their own homes or in facilities, e.g., nursing facilities, group homes, etc. All supplies and equipment needed for the alleviation or prevention of distressing symptoms related to the terminal illness should be made available to patients. Programs should establish parameters for blood transfusions, laboratory tests, and medications that ensure appropriate care and use of services. No treatment should be automatically excluded. Patients should have 24-hour-a-day access to medications.
- **Hospice programs have an organized governing body** that has complete and ultimate responsibility for the organization. The hospice governing body entrusts the hospice administrator with overall management responsibility for operating the hospice, including planning, organizing, staffing, and evaluating the organization and its services.
- **Hospice is committed to continuous assessment and improvement** of the quality and efficiency of its services.

Adapted from *Standards of a Hospice Program of Care.* Arlington, Virginia: National Hospice Organization; 1993. National Hospice Organization. Hospice services guidelines and definitions. *Hospice J.* 1996;11(2):65–73.

# Roles of Physicians Practicing Hospice/Palliative Medicine

In hospice/palliative care settings, treatment decisions are inextricably linked to the physician's primary task, which is helping patients to choose the best interventions for specific situations and then providing the best possible care.[19,20] Dr. Saunders reminds physicians that "Appropriate treatment for a patient need not include every effort to prolong life regardless of its quality, and what could be done for a patient with an acute remediable condition may be burdensome for one who is terminally ill."[21]

Table 7 describes several roles of physicians who practice hospice/palliative medicine. Dying patients look to physicians not only for diagnosis and treatment, but also for reassurance, guidance, and a renewed sense of hope. Most patients believe that physicians have a duty to help to alleviate their suffering regardless of its cause.They want physicians to care about them, to know what they value, to treat them with dignity and respect, to view them as human beings who exist apart from their disease, and to ease their suffering.[22] For more information about the roles of physicians associated with hospice/palliative care programs, see *UNIPAC Five: Caring for the Terminally Ill—Communication and the Physician's Role on the Interdisciplinary Team.*

## Table 7: Roles of Physicians Practicing Hospice/Palliative Medicine

**Care for Patients**

- Provide guidance and support as patients make the transition from curative to palliative care
- Provide competent assessments and diagnoses
- Provide information about diagnosis, prognosis, and treatment options
- Provide guidance during the process of making treatment decisions
- Respect the patient's beliefs, values, and goals
- Provide skilled, effective interventions that meet the patient's needs
- Collaborate with the patient's attending physician and, in hospice settings, with members of the interdisciplinary team to achieve outcomes that meet the patient's needs
- Offer caring presence
- Support the patient's search for a renewed sense of meaning, purpose, and hope
- Serve as an advocate to help patients to receive needed services
- Participate in teaching and research activities to improve the standard of patient care

**Care for Family Members**

- Provide guidance and support as families make the transition from curative to palliative goals for continued care
- Provide information about diagnosis, prognosis, and treatment options
- Provide guidance during the process of making treatment decisions so that the patient's wishes are honored
- Adjust therapies to meet the capabilities of family members and teach patient care techniques
- Provide ongoing emotional support and reassurance

**Care for Self**

- Attain professional competence
- Seek peer support
- Learn stress management techniques and practice self-care activities, including taking time for exercise, interaction with family members, and vacations

**Care for the Team**

- Participate in team meetings and listen respectfully to help to develop mutual trust and respect
- Ask for help from team members

(*Continued*)

- Serve as a resource to improve the team's medical skills
- Pay attention and learn from other team members
- Help the team to stay focused on the patient's and family's problems
- Watch for signs of exhaustion and stress in self and other team members

**Care for the Organization**

- Demonstrate careful stewardship of the organization's resources to improve patient access to needed care
- Participate in quality-improvement activities
- Help with administrative tasks as appropriate
- Assist management in focusing resources where they are most needed to alleviate the patient's and family's suffering
- Promote humane and efficient management strategies that reduce staff turnover and improve patient outcomes

## Physicians as Healers

One goal of hospice/palliative medicine is to help patients and family members reestablish a sense of hope, meaning, and purpose. Expectations that physicians will treat not only the patient's disease but also will care for the person who is experiencing illness, have their roots in ancient mythology. In the oldest known version of a common myth, Asklepios was a physician, half-god and half-man, whose skills were the basis of Greek and Roman medical traditions for nearly 2000 years:[23]

> Apollo, the god of healing, consorted with a mortal woman, who, in accordance with her father's demands, married another mortal instead of the god. In a fit of jealous rage, Apollo had the woman killed. As she was burning on her funeral pyre, Apollo first cut his child out of the woman's womb, then named the boy Asklepios and took him to Chiron, the Centaur. Chiron raised Asklepios and taught him the art of healing. Asklepios was so skilled as a physician and healer he was able to cure illness, alleviate suffering, prevent some people from dying, and raise the dead. Fearful that this half-god, half-mortal might usurp the power of the gods, Zeus struck Asklepios with a thunderbolt and killed him.[23]

Over the centuries, the myth evolved to meet changing cultural and political needs, but the essence of the myth remained: Asklepios was a compassionate healer, who was revered because he cared so deeply about humankind that he was willing to risk death to alleviate the suffering of all who came his way, regardless of their station in life. According to later versions of the myth, Asklepios rose from the dead and ascended to heaven, where he continued to heal those who prayed to him. The commonly quoted 16th century adage echoes the Asklepian myth: "To cure sometimes, to relieve often, to comfort always."[24]

# Roles of Patients at the End of Life

As medical advances prolong the process of dying, the role of a terminally ill patient has become more complex. Everyone involved—patient, family member, and healthcare professional—struggles with the challenging task of envisioning meaningful roles for a person who is dying, but may continue living for many months.[25]

When terminally ill patients know that their physical symptoms will be controlled and that they will not be abandoned by their family and physician, they may experience a sense of increased satisfaction, completion, and personal growth as their lives draw to a close.[26] The activities listed in Table 8 have been described as the *developmental tasks* of the dying. The tasks can provide patients with meaningful roles that strengthen their bonds with friends and family members. The tasks also can support a profound sense of meaning during the final stages of living.[8] However, care must to taken to avoid placing additional burdens on profoundly ill patients by insisting that they engage in specific activities. (See *UNIPAC Two: Alleviating Psychological and Spiritual Pain in the Terminally Ill.*)

**Table 8: Developmental Tasks of People Who Are Dying[8]**

**Develop a Renewed Sense of Personhood and Meaning**

- Find meanings for life through life review and personal narrative
- Develop a sense of worthiness, both in the past and in the current situation
- Learn to accept love and caring from other people

**Bring Closure to Personal and Community Relationships**

- Say good-bye to family members and friends with expressions of regret, gratitude, appreciation, and affection
- Ask for and grant forgiveness to estranged friends and family members so that reconciliation can occur
- Say good-bye to community relationships (employment, civic, and religious organizations) with expressions of regret, gratitude, forgiveness, and appreciation

**Bring Closure to Worldly Affairs**

- Arrange for the transfer of fiscal, legal, and social responsibilities

**Accept the Finality of Life and Surrender to the Transcendent**

- Express the depth of personal tragedy that dying may represent and acknowledge the totality of personal loss
- Withdraw from the world and accept increased dependency
- Develop a sense of awe and accept the seeming chaos that can precede transcendence

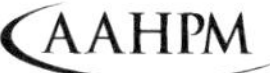

# Roles of Family Members

When one family member becomes terminally ill, the entire family system is thrown out of balance and must adapt to changing conditions. The stresses associated with adapting to the difficult challenges of a terminal illness may trigger or exacerbate long-standing family problems, including differences of opinion about family rules, roles, and beliefs. For more information about family systems, see *UNIPAC Five: Caring for the Terminally Ill—Communication and the Physician's Role on the Interdisciplinary Team.* Table 9 describes several family roles that can help patients to achieve the developmental tasks of the dying.

**Table 9: Role of the Family When One Member Is Dying**

- Help the dying person remain as independent as possible for as long as possible
- Help steward the financial and human resources of the dying person and the family to best achieve the patient's goals
- Allow the dying person to die in the place of his or her own choosing, whenever feasible
- Work with members of a hospice/palliative interdisciplinary team to identify interventions that will improve the quality of life of the patient and family as much as possible
- Call for help when the dying person is in distress and/or the family is exhausted
- Express as much love, caring, and forgiveness as possible so that the dying person will feel free to do the same

# Components of Beneficial Physician/Patient Relationships

The components of beneficial physician–patient relationships have been described in several models of patient care, some of which propose patient autonomy as an alternative to medical paternalism. Most models pay insufficient attention to the many-layered and sometimes conflicting aspects of therapeutic physician–patient relationships.[27] In an effort to include the best features of both medical paternalism and patient autonomy, Thomasma proposed a *physician conscience* model based on the rules of prudent judgment. See Table 10.

## Table 10: Physician Conscience Model of Patient Care: Rules for Making Prudent Judgments[27]

- **Both the physician and the patient must feel free to make informed decisions.** Physicians and patients must feel free to express their beliefs and values about treatments without fear of coercion. Physicians often refrain from expressing their own views about treatments for fear of influencing patients or inadvertently coercing them into making certain decisions. However, most patients want guidance from physicians when making decisions about the benefits and burdens of treatment options. If physicians abandon their role as guides, who will fill it?
- **Physicians are morally required to pay increased attention to patient vulnerability.** The inherent imbalance of power in patient–physician relationships requires almost excessive attention to treating patients with dignity and respect. Vulnerable patients should be treated with increased caring, not disdain.
- **Physicians must use their power responsibly to care for the patient.** Because illness assaults personal integrity and increases a patient's sense of vulnerability, physicians should restore the balance of power as much as possible by encouraging patient autonomy.
- **Physicians must have integrity.** Physicians must respect a patient's values, cultural beliefs and religious traditions. Some characteristics of moral and medical judgment apply to all physicians. Physicians should learn the skills involved in making prudent judgments in the context of a specific situation.
- **Physicians must have a healthy respect for moral ambiguity.** Physician training focuses on problem solving and clinical closure, but most contemporary moral debates have no right or wrong answer for every situation. Respect for ambiguity, characteristic of a mature mind, allows physicians to rationally discuss alternatives without succumbing to the need to be right or to impose personal values on patients and family members.

*Hospice is a place of meeting. Physical and spiritual, doing and accepting, giving and receiving, all have to be brought together . . . the dying need the community, its help and fellowship . . . the community needs the dying to make it think of eternal issues and to make it listen . . . we are debtors to those who can make us learn such things as to be gentle and to approach others with true attention and respect.*

— DR. CICELY SAUNDERS, (quoted by Stoddard[1])

## Origins of Hospice/Palliative Care

Romans used the Latin root word, *hospes* to describe both hosts and guests, a usage that emphasized the subtle relationships connecting both parties.[1] The Latin root word for hospice, *hospitium*, referred to a place where guests were received with hospitality and lodging, concepts associated with several modern words, including hospice, hostel, hotel, and hospital.[28]

Dr. Balfour Mount coined the term, *palliative care*, from the Latin root word, *pallium*, which referred to an outer garment that covered or cloaked a person or object. The Latin derivation suggests that palliative care can effectively cloak the symptoms of terminal illness. The ancient Indo-European word, *pelte*, has been suggested as an additional etymological root for palliative care, because it implies an increasingly active role for physicians who practice palliative medicine.[29] *Pelte* referred to a hide or skin stretched over a frame and used to shield or protect something. *Pelte* suggests that skilled palliative medicine physicians offer interventions that help to protect and shield patients from the devastating effects of terminal illness, while assisting them in their search for hope, purpose, and meaning.

## Early Hospice Movement

### Development of Early Hospices

The roots of the hospice movement began long ago. As early as 2500 BCE, healers in India and Egypt developed institutions for medical education and health care.[28] In the 6th century BCE, Buddhists established a network of medical centers across India.[30] The Greeks and Romans often diagnosed and cared for the sick and dying in religious temples. In 475 CE, Fabiola, a Roman matron, opened a refuge for travelers, the sick, and the dying.

During the Middle Ages, Christian religious orders established networks of hospices across Europe, in particular along the routes of the Crusades. The hospices provided refuges for weary travelers, for pilgrims in search of spiritual renewal, and for people who were dying. Hospices offered hospitality, including care for the body and respect for the soul as people journeyed either from one place to another or from this life to the next.[31] When a series of plagues in the 14th century decimated the population of Europe, killing more than 25 million people, widespread societal disruption left the sick and the dying with no one else to help them.[28]

# Modern Hospice Movement

## Development of Hospices in Europe

In the 1600s, Vincent de Paul, a French priest and former slave, founded a nursing order called the Sisters of Charity, which devoted itself to caring for the sick and dying.[32] In 1879, Sister Mary Aikenhead, of the Irish Sisters of Charity, founded Our Lady's Hospice in Dublin.[33,34] In 1891, the Anglican Sisters of the Society of St. Margaret opened the Hostel of God, which continues to care for critically ill patients in London to this day. In 1905, the Irish Sisters of Charity founded St. Joseph's Hospice in the East End of London, where the modern hospice movement began with the work of Dr. Cicely Saunders.[31]

### Dr. Cicely Saunders

Dr. Saunders is usually credited with developing the art and science of modern hospice care. She established physician training programs to improve competence in palliative medicine and formulated the basic principles of hospice care, which include vigilant attention to the details of patient care and careful research to support claims about an intervention's effectiveness (see Table 3, page 20).

Dr. Saunders began her career as a nurse and social worker. Her overriding concern was alleviating the suffering of dying patients. After completing her medical training, Dr. Saunders became the first full-time medical director at St. Joseph's, where she pioneered the use of oral opioids to control pain and developed the concept of *total pain* to describe the all-encompassing physical, emotional, spiritual, and social distress experienced by many dying patients. While caring for David Tasma, a dying Polish Jew from the Warsaw ghetto, Dr. Saunders described her vision of care for terminally ill patients. Tasma replied, "I want what is in your mind and your heart" and donated £500 so that he could be a "window" in her new hospice home. In 1967, Dr. Saunders opened the world-renowned St. Christopher's Hospice in Sydenham (south London), which continues to focus on alleviating physical, emotional, spiritual, and social contributors to total pain.[35]

## Development of Hospices in the United States

### Dr. Elizabeth Kübler-Ross

During the same period that Dr. Saunders was developing the principles of hospice care, Elizabeth Kübler-Ross, MD (a Swiss-born psychiatrist who emigrated to the United States), was interviewing terminally ill patients about their reactions to dying. In 1969, she published *On Death and Dying*,[36] which rapidly became a best-seller and sparked widespread interest in the care of dying patients. In her book, Dr. Kübler-Ross described both the conspiracy of silence that surrounds terminally ill patients and five common stages or reactions to dying: denial, anger, bargaining, depression, and acceptance. Although Kübler-Ross used the term *stages of dying*, she did not mean to imply that all patients experience the same five reactions in exactly the same order.

## Organizational Models of Hospice Care in the United States

Hospice care has been one of the fastest growing social and medical movements in the United States. The first hospice program opened in 1974. By 2000, approximately 3,100 programs were caring for 700,000 patients.[37]

Several models of hospice care evolved in the United States to meet differing community needs; some are free-standing entities (37%) and some are affiliated with hospitals (35%), home health agencies (22%), and hospital systems (9%). The remaining (6%) are under other auspices. All Medicare-certified hospice programs must provide the same services whether they are community based or operated by other entities. (For a description of required services, see Table 20, page 61.)

Originally, most hospice programs were incorporated as nonprofit organizations, but ownership trends are changing. In 2000, 73% were nonprofit, 20% were for-profit, and 7% were operated by the government. Ninety-one percent of hospices are Medicare certified and 55% are accredited.[37]

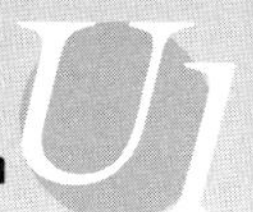

*End-of-life care should be viewed as an integral part of the continuum of care provided by the health care system.*

—Cassel and Vladeck[38]

*A medicine that embodies an acceptance of death would represent a great change in the common conception, and might set the stage for viewing the care of dying people not as an afterthought when all else has failed but as one of the ends of medicine. The goal of a peaceful death should be as much a part of the purpose of medicine as the promotion of good heath. That means medicine must abandon the modern cultic myth that in the cure of disease lies the cure of death. . . . Disease and death will have their day.*

—Daniel Callahan, adapted from *The Troubled Dream of Life*[39]

## Locations and Causes of Death

Since the 1940s, the locations and causes of death in the United States have changed dramatically. Before the advent of antibiotics and advanced technologies, people usually died in their homes over the course of a few days or weeks. Now most people die in institutions. Of the approximately 2.5 million people who die annually in the United States,[40] more than three-quarters die in institutions: 61% in hospitals and 17% in nursing facilities.[40]

The prevalence of chronic illnesses has altered the usual process of dying, which has become so prolonged that it is often recognized as a distinct stage of life, much like childhood, adolescence, and adulthood. Society continues to struggle with the challenging task of providing cost-effective, high-quality, compassionate care for the increasing numbers of patients whose deaths occur after months of gradual debilitation due to illnesses such as cancer, end-stage renal disease, arteriosclerotic diseases, and Alzheimer's disease.

## Barriers to Effective End-of-Life Care

Despite a substantial increase in societal concern about end-of-life care, there is no clear indication that the care of dying patients has improved.[41] In the United States, the emphasis on *curegiving* rather than *caregiving* continues to foster intensive and sometimes futile therapy in an effort to ward off death. When death becomes inevitable, despite all medical efforts to the contrary, physicians often refer patients to other caregivers due to the misconception that "*there is nothing more I can do.*"[42] Barriers to effective end-of life care include those listed in Table 11.

**Table 11: Barriers to Effective End-of-Life Care**

- The mistaken, widespread belief among physicians that they have nothing further to offer dying patients[43]
- The widespread, often unconscious perception that a patient's death is due to physician failure
- Misconceptions about hospice/palliative medicine, e.g., the work is depressing and lacks professional satisfaction
- Misconceptions about palliative medicine interventions on the part of many healthcare professionals, e.g., effective interventions are lacking and the use of opioids causes addiction[44]
- The absence of palliative medicine in most medical school curricula and a lack of hospice/palliative care mentors and training for healthcare professionals at all educational levels
- Lack of practical formats for transmitting information about hospice/palliative medicine to medical students and attending physicians[45]
- Lack of academic medical center focus on research and clinical issues related to palliative care and lack of skilled faculty to teach hospice/palliative medicine

Expert pain management is central to the provision of effective end-of-life care, but studies document the continued inadequacy of pain management in the United States. In 1994, the United States Department of Health and Human Services published the *Clinical Practice Guidelines No 9: Management of Cancer Pain* to help to educate physicians about effective pain management techniques.[46]

In 1995, the results of the multistate SUPPORT study indicated that most terminally ill patients continued to die alone and in pain and, in many cases, experienced needless suffering due to poor communication about end-of-life care issues.[47]

In 1997, the Institute of Medicine (IOM) report, *Approaching Death: Improving Care at the End of Life*, concluded that, despite the availability of effective options for relieving most pain, many dying people suffer needlessly from serious pain and other distressing symptoms that clinicians could prevent or relieve with existing knowledge and therapies. Patients suffer from errors of omission and commission, resulting in under- and overtreatment that prolongs their suffering.[44]

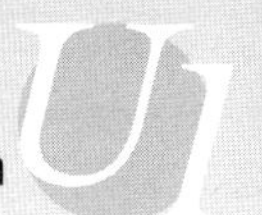

Like many other organizations, the American Medical Association (AMA) now recognizes system-wide deficiencies in end-of-life care and recommends increased emphasis on palliation to improve the system's ability to care for terminally ill patients.[48]

# Models for Integrating Hospice/Palliative Care into the Healthcare System

## Suggested Organization Model

Effective healthcare systems provide a continuum of services that meet peoples' needs from birth through death. In response to concerns about the limited role hospice/palliative care plays in the current healthcare system, several organizations have proposed models to expand the role of palliative care.[9] See Figure 1 for a suggested model for palliative care services.

## Victoria Model

Downing, Braithwaite, and Wilde propose a broad role for palliative care.[49] Their model, developed for the Victoria Hospice Society, is described in Figures 2, 3, and 4 and in Tables 12, 13, and 14. The Victoria model of palliative care encompasses a wide range of services, which offer alternatives both to curative care and to euthanasia. See Figure 2 and Table 12 for descriptions of the proposed spectrum of palliative care.

**Figure 1:** Suggested Model of Palliative Care Services

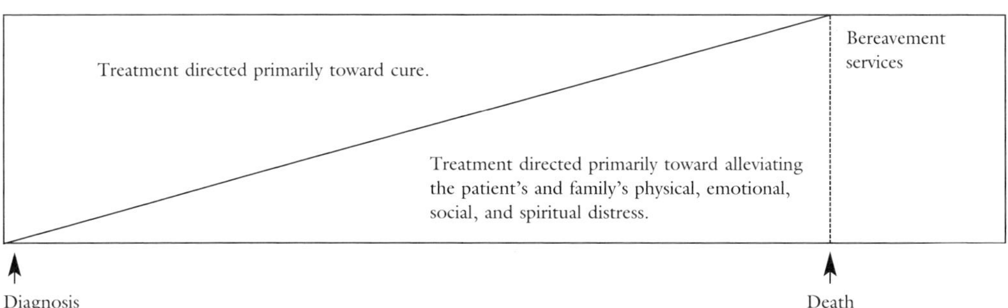


*Cancer Pain Relief and Palliative Care.* Technical Report Series 804. Geneva: World Health Organization; 1990. Figure 3:16. Figure modified and reprinted with permission from the World Health Organization.

## Table 12: The Victoria Model for Integrating Palliative Care into the Healthcare System: The Spectrum of Care[47]

- **Acute care** (black) appears on the left of the continuum. It focuses on cure and the extension of life and includes highly aggressive treatments. Acute care treatments may result in symptom relief within days, weeks, or months, but the emphasis is on cure.
- **Palliative care** (blue, green, and yellow) comprises the middle of the continuum. It focuses on palliation of symptoms and improved quality of life. Palliative care includes a wide range of interventions, from oral medications to surgery. Palliative treatments are categorized as active (blue), comfort (green), or urgent (yellow), but a combined approach often is necessary. In any case, adequate symptom relief should be achieved within hours, or days at the most. Urgent palliative care should result in full comfort within hours.
- **Euthanasia** (red) is on the far right of the continuum. Because the intent of euthanasia and physician-assisted suicide is cessation of life, it is not part of the continuum of palliative interventions.

**Figure 2:** The Spectrum of Palliative Care

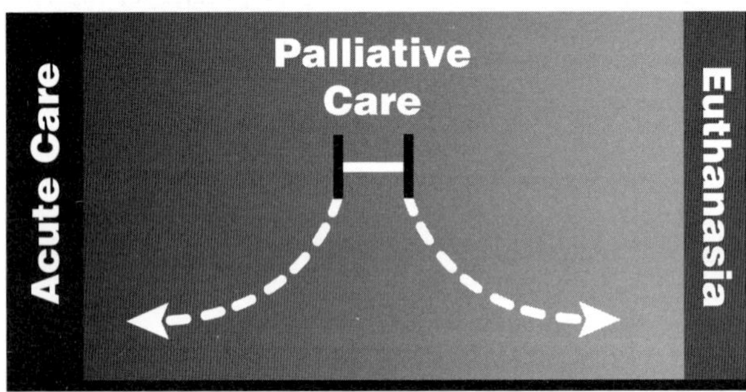


Figure adapted with permission from the *Journal of Palliative Care*. Downing MC, Braithwaite DL, Wilde JM. Victoria BGY palliative care model—a new model for the 1990s. *J Palliat Care* 1993;9(4);2632.

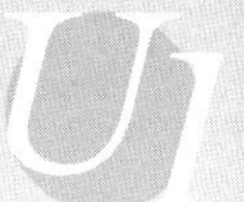

### Three Forms of Palliative Care

Table 13 describes three forms of palliative care included in the Victoria Model. In the model, the continuum of palliative treatments is dynamic: patients move from active palliation to comfort palliation to urgent palliation and back again, depending on the situation. For example, a shift to urgent palliation may be necessary to control emerging new symptoms, sudden complications, or severe distress. After symptoms are controlled, a return to comfort palliation may adequately maintain the patient's comfort. To fully meet the needs of terminally ill patients, programs must skillfully provide the entire continuum of palliative services. If programs cannot provide effective interventions, physician-assisted suicide and euthanasia will continue to gain support.

**Table 13: The Victoria Model: Three Forms of Palliative Care[49]**

- **Active palliation** (blue): Active palliation includes active investigations and aggressive treatments that modify the disease. Treatments are not aimed at extending life, but extension may occur. Examples of active palliation include chemotherapy, hormonal therapy, aggressive antibiotic therapy, cerebral irradiation, and steroids, all of which offer symptom relief, but may also prolong life. Active palliative treatments can be invasive and usually require inpatient care or repeated office visits. If complications arise, they are usually treated actively.
- **Comfort palliation** (green): Most terminally ill patients live and die comfortably with comfort palliation. Interventions are noninvasive and include drug and adjuvant measures to relieve symptoms, not to modify the disease. Prolonged life is not intended, but may occur due to adequate symptom relief and emotional support. Drug therapies include strong opioids, major tranquilizers, antidepressants, NSAIDs, steroids, etc. Other interventions include relaxation and diversion, short-term psychotherapy, grief counseling, and spiritual support that focuses on renewing the patient's sense of purpose, meaning, and hope. Most care is provided at home, although some inpatient care or respite care may be needed. Complications usually are treated with noninvasive palliative interventions.
- **Urgent palliation** (yellow): Urgent palliation is necessary when symptom emergencies occur, when patients experience moderate to severe symptoms, and when sudden complications arise. Urgent palliation relieves symptoms within a few hours so that patients do not endure uncontrolled symptoms for days or weeks at a time or die with uncontrolled pain. Interventions are aggressive and often rely on subcutaneous or intravenous (IV) routes. Medications include potent opioids, anxiolytics, tranquilizers, etc. Dosages may be much higher than many physicians usually prescribe and are rapidly titrated to relieve symptoms as quickly as possible. When comfort is achieved, dosages remain constant or are titrated down, as long as comfort is maintained. When urgent palliation is used effectively, patients rarely experience a crescendo of pain toward the end of life. If uncontrolled symptoms do appear as death approaches, urgent palliation is mandatory. Sedation may be necessary to achieve relief. Urgent care requires experience, skill, judgment, and courage. It often requires inpatient care, but may be provided in the home setting with continuous supervision and support. Shortened life is not the intent of urgent palliative care, but it may occur.

**Figure 3:** Life Promotion–Death Acceptance Tension in Palliative Care

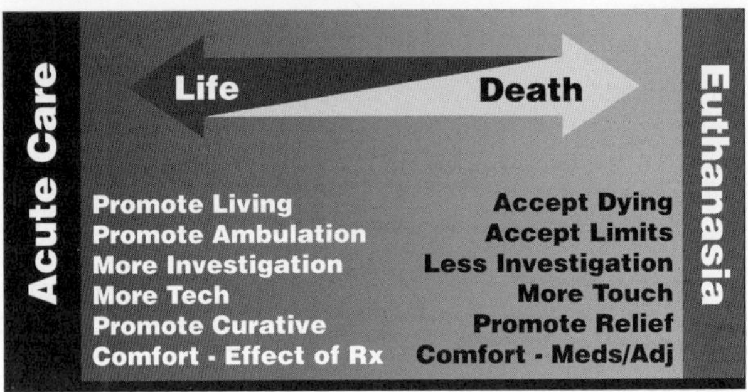


Figure adapted with permission from the *Journal of Palliative Care.* Downing MC, Braithwaite DL, Wilde JM. Victoria BGY palliative care model—a new model for the 1990s. *J Palliat Care* 1993;9(4);2632.

## Tensions Inherent in Palliative Care

See Figures 3 and 4 and Table 14 for descriptions of tensions experienced by everyone involved with palliative care, including patients, family members, and healthcare professionals.

**Figure 4:** Emotional Tension in Palliative Care

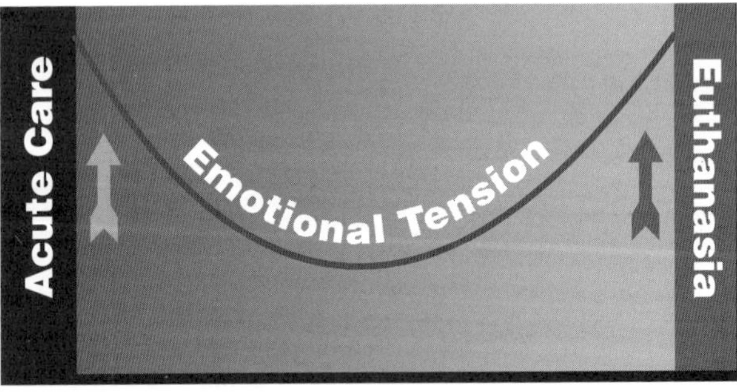


Figure adapted with permission from the *Journal of Palliative Care.* Downing MC, Braithwaite DL, Wilde JM. Victoria BGY palliative care model—a new model for the 1990s. *J Palliat Care* 1993;9(4);2632.

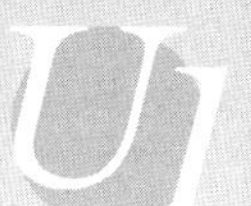

## Table 14: Tensions Inherent in Palliative Care[49]

- **Tension between Life Promotion and Death Acceptance.** The dynamic tension between life promotion and death acceptance is normal and often continues until death. Examples of life-promoting behaviors and attitudes include the desire to continue living, to find a cure, to remain active as long as possible, to order tests to see if something can be corrected, to eat and drink, and to remain mentally clear. Examples of death acceptance include thinking or talking about dying, promoting comfort rather than cure, recognizing limits, and feeling as if life has been lived long enough. The natural tension between life promotion and death acceptance often results in conflict among involved parties. For example, a patient may be inwardly preparing to die while the physician and family are focusing on life-promoting behaviors, such as eating and drinking. Later, the patient may experience a shift toward more life-promoting behaviors just as the physician and family experience a shift toward death acceptance.
- **Emotional Tension.** Emotional tension is most pronounced during the active and urgent forms of palliative care. When patients move from acute care to active palliative care, stress increases as patients, physicians, and family members question whether continued active treatment is in the patient's best interests. The least amount of stress tends to occur in the middle of the spectrum—comfort palliation—because the goals of treatment are clear and treatment is fairly straightforward. Stress increases when patients require urgent palliative care. Many physicians are reluctant to use the dosages of medication necessary to control severe symptoms due to their concerns about hastening death. Additional stress occurs if symptoms remain uncontrolled or patients request physician-assisted suicide or euthanasia.

# Hospice/Palliative Medicine in the Home Care Setting

When asked, most people indicate they would prefer to die at home, but few patients see that wish fulfilled.[50] A 1996 Gallup Organization survey revealed that almost nine out of ten Americans (88%) would prefer to receive care and ultimately die in their own home (or in the home of a family member) if they were terminally ill and had 6 months or less to live.[51] Despite the widespread desire to die at home, the percentage of home deaths in developed countries has declined rapidly, to about 15% in North America.[52] Among hospice patients the trend is reversing. In 1995, 77% of hospice patients in the United States died in their own homes, 19% died in an institutional facility, and 4% died in other settings.[37] For nonhospice patients, factors contributing to the increase in institutionalized death include the following:[50]

- The medicalization of dying
- Disproportionate funding for hospital services at the expense of hospice and home care services
- Few physicians are willing to make home visits, which means that hospitals may be the only place where physicians are available to care for seriously ill patients.
- The widespread perception that hospitals are places where cures are possible and excellent services are available, which may be true for acutely ill patients, but is less true for most terminally ill patients
- Wider use of parenteral opioids in hospital settings, even though adequate amounts of opioids are rarely used

The benefits of hospice/palliative care in the home setting include the following:

- Increased patient and family control of medical care
- Familiar surroundings for the patient, e.g., home, bed, pillow, and food
- Decreased isolation and better access to family members, friends, and pets
- No need to observe visiting hours
- Less exposure to iatrogenic infections
- Less expense if family members provide most of the care
- Increased access to work-related activities, hobbies, and nature

# Barriers to Effective Hospice/Palliative Care in the Home Setting

In the United States, the majority of terminally ill patients either are not referred for hospice care or are referred so late in the course of their illness they cannot take full advantage of hospice services.[53] Doyle[50] describes several barriers to effective home care, including those listed in Table 15. In the United States, geographic separation of families and lack of insurance coverage pose particular problems.

**Table 15: Barriers to Effective Hospice/Palliative Care in the Home Setting[50]**

**Lack of Effective Management of Pain and Other Symptoms**

- Poor physician skills in managing pain, particularly in the home setting, e.g., in one study only 19% of family physicians were prescribing opioids[54]
- Physician misconceptions about opioids and fears of legal reprisals if adequate dosages of opioids are prescribed
- Patient/family misconceptions about opioids and fears of addiction
- See *UNIPAC Three: Assessment and Treatment of Pain in the Terminally Ill*

**Lack of Effective Management of Psychological, Spiritual, and Social Pain**

- Insufficient physician training on palliative care in the home setting[55]
- Lack of physician training on recognizing and providing effective interventions for psychological, spiritual, and social pain
- Lack of skill and effective teamwork when caring for patients and families whose belief systems contribute to suffering
- Patient and family reluctance to voice concerns about dying, social isolation, and loneliness
- Fear of the unknown and of dying in physical pain and emotional distress
- Fear of becoming a burden to family members and relying on family members for enemas, suppositories, and cleaning soiled bed linens
- See *UNIPAC Two: Alleviating Psychological and Spiritual Pain in the Terminally Ill*

(*Continued*)

**Lack of Adequate Communication**

- Physician—lack of physician training in communication
- Patient—concerns about upsetting the family
- Family— concerns about "bothering" busy physicians with what may be construed as minor problems
- See *UNIPAC Five: Caring for the Terminally Ill—Communication and the Physician's Role on the Interdisciplinary Team*

**Lack of Family Help and Support**

- Prevalence of dual-career families and geographical separation
- Lack of acknowledgment of the family's suffering
- Lack of emotional support and education about symptoms and interventions
- Lack of periodic relief from caregiving responsibilities
- Lack of understanding about hospice care so that referrals are not requested

**Lack of Adequate Planning**

- Need to provide and maintain supplies and durable medical equipment in the home
- Need to coordinate financial benefits
- Need to anticipate crises and prepare patients and families for problems such as eating difficulties, progressive weakness, incontinence, constipation, hypercalcemia, and increasing edema

**Lack of Adequate Coordination**

- Need for timely home visits by physicians, nurses, social workers, clergy, and home health aides
- Need for availability of medications
- Need for delivery of durable medical equipment, such as special mattresses, hospital beds, bedside commodes, wheel chairs
- Need for temporary transfers for inpatient care

**Lack of Insurance Coverage for Home Care and Inadequate Reimbursement for Healthcare Professionals**

- Inadequate coverage of oral medications in home settings (many insurance policies provide more coverage for invasive interventions in inpatient settings)
- Inadequate coverage for intensive palliative treatments in the home setting
- Inadequate reimbursement for home care visits, which may involve significant time and travel, especially in rural settings

# Home Visits by Physicians

Terminally ill patients receiving hospice/palliative care place high value on home visits by physicians. When focus groups of current hospice patients and family members were asked to rank the importance of hospice services, they consistently ranked physician home visits second in importance only to visits by home health aides.[56]

The value of physician home visits cannot be overemphasized. Unless physicians make home visits, they are unlikely to gain full understanding of the patient's and family's concerns as they struggle to cope with extremely difficult circumstances. During the course of home visits, physicians have the opportunity to:

- Meet the family members who are caring for the patient
- Tailor therapies to meet the functional abilities of patients and family members
- Discuss, in a more relaxed setting, the patient's diagnosis and prognosis, family concerns about the costs of treatment, and the patient's and family's values and beliefs
- Explore the family's concerns about fulfilling promises to the patient, e.g., "We will take care of you at home and never send you to a nursing home"
- Explore the best alternatives if a promise becomes impossible to keep
- Help family members cope with feelings of guilt about their inability to keep a promise

Indications for physician home visits include the following:[57]

- The patient is terminally ill and wishes to die at home
- Evaluate suspected caregiver burnout
- Suspected psychosocial problems
- Need to provide patient and family with reassurance
- Family conference
- Patient living alone, especially if recently bereaved or separated
- Mental impairment
- Major mobility problems
- History of falling or accidents

- Imminent institutionalization
- Recent hospital discharge, especially if recovery was incomplete

## Assessments in the Home

During home visits, physicians should make physical and environmental assessments, review the patient's functional status and use of medications, and assess the patient's and family's need for additional services and assistance.[57] See Table 16 for descriptions of assessments.

### Table 16: Assessments by Physicians in Home Settings

**Environmental assessment.** Home assessments are more likely to reveal situations such as the following:

- ***Safety.*** Patients with unsteady gait, lack of hand rails, particularly in stair wells, stairs between the patient's bedroom and bathroom, loose carpet, forgetful patients in homes with gas stoves, paranoid patients with guns in the home, etc.
- ***Independence vs. privacy:*** The patient's need to dress and toilet in private and to spend time alone may conflict with the family's need to monitor the patient's safety and prevent falls, ensure appropriate use of medications, etc. The patient's desire for independence and privacy should be honored as much as possible.
- ***Staff safety.*** Some homes are located in unsafe areas. Security escorts may be needed; visits by members of the interdisciplinary team may need to be made in twos, especially at night.

**Patient assessment.** Home visits can provide important information about the following symptoms:

- Incontinence may be determined by odor; it may result from lack of easy access to a toilet.
- Cachexia may be related to a lack of palatable food.
- Depression may be related to dark rooms, loneliness, stressful family interactions, or immobility.
- Constipation may be due to refusal to take laxatives to decrease the burden of care on stressed family members.

**Family assessment.** Family assessments are crucial to determine the family's ability to assist with the patient's therapy.

- Attentive, capable, well-rested families can better manage around-the-clock medication schedules.
- Patients left alone for long periods of time may benefit from long-acting or sustained-release medications.
- Very distressed and disorganized families may require more frequent nursing visits to replace transdermal patches and/or refill carefully labeled pill containers.
- Respite care may be needed to relieve family members of caregiving responsibilities.

# Management of Specific Symptoms in the Home Setting

Even very difficult symptoms often can be managed in the home setting by using effective doses of appropriate medications and alternative delivery routes. Some symptoms are particularly troublesome to manage at home, not because they are medically complicated, but because they are malodorous, are frightening for laypeople, or require family involvement in the patient's personal care. Doyle describes several symptoms that may be troublesome to manage in the home setting, including those listed in Table 17.[50] For more information about managing difficult symptoms, see *UNIPAC Two: Alleviating Psychological and Spiritual Pain in the Terminally Ill*, *UNIPAC Three: Assessment and Treatment of Pain in the Terminally Ill*, and *UNIPAC Four: Management of Selected Nonpain Symptoms in the Terminally Ill.*

**Table 17: Suggestions for Managing Specific Symptoms in the Home Setting[50]**

**Insomnia**

- Anxiety often increases as death approaches. Sleeping difficulties at night are common. If families are expected to provide patient care, they must be allowed to rest. Concerted effort must be made to ensure that both patients and family members sleep well at night.
- Reschedule laxatives, diuretics, or stimulants such as albuterol so that patients and families can sleep.
- Use more sedating antidepressants and anticonvulsants at bedtime.
- Because opioid requirements often are higher at night, slow-release products can be quite useful. To help patients get 8 hours of uninterrupted sleep, immediate-release opioid doses can usually be doubled at bedtime, and the infusion rate of continuous infusions of opioids often can be doubled at night.
- If bad dreams or delusions interfere with sleep, major tranquilizers such as thioridazine (Mellaril) or chlorpromazine (Thorazine) may be more useful than benzodiazepine hypnotics.

**Fecal Incontinence**

- This symptom may not be medically complicated, but it often contributes disproportionately to a patient's suffering because it results in further loss of privacy and the need to rely on family members for very personal care. Emotional distress due to fecal incontinence may cause patients and/or family members to request the patient's transfer to an institutional setting. In some cases, fecal incontinence symbolizes a final loss of independence and results in requests for physician-assisted suicide.
- Acknowledge that fecal incontinence is common, as is the embarrassment associated with it.

(*Continued*)

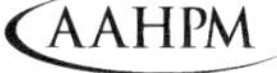

- Carefully evaluate the patient's diet, medications, and toileting history; they may reveal treatable causes.
- Consider the risk of fecal incontinence before prescribing osmotic laxatives like lactulose and sorbitol that often cause loose stools.
- Develop a toileting schedule.
- Schedule use of suppositories or enemas to clear bowels.
- Teach pain management techniques, transfer techniques, and use of a bedside commode.
- Provide patient and family education about skin care, diet, laxatives, deodorizing techniques, and privacy.

**Convulsions**

- Convulsions are very frightening for patients and family members, but usually can be managed at home with rectal diazepam or subcutaneous midazolam.
- Teach families to administer needed medication.
- Prevent convulsions with prophylactic use of oral anticonvulsants. If swallowing is too difficult, use SC phenobarbital or fosphenytoin, or teach family members to use rectal mini-enemas of valproate. Achieve recommended serum levels of anticonvulsants when possible.

**Hemorrhage from Any Site**

- The sight of blood usually frightens patients and family members regardless of its medical significance.
- If bleeding is likely, avoid NSAIDs, Coumadin, heparin, and other drugs that may cause bleeding.
- Consider treatments designed to control bleeding, e.g., amino caproic acid or radiation therapy.
- Control hypertension aggressively and change dressings over tumors or deep wounds with great care and as infrequently as practical.
- Provide patient and family education, and keep special supplies on hand, such as red or dark brown towels.
- Make careful plans to manage future bleeding with compression, gel foam, or fibrin powder.
- If a hemorrhage is slow and the patient is ambulatory and mentally clear, transfer to a hospice/palliative care inpatient unit or an emergency center may be warranted. Nasal or vaginal packing or even an arterial embolization may provide important additional weeks of life. Extra nursing visits are necessary, and a compromise is usually necessary between optimal cleanliness and increased bleeding risks. The primary risk of visits to an emergency room is dying in an intensive care unit.
- If massive bleeding is likely to cause a patient's death, make detailed plans to deal with an emergency situation to avoid crises and last-minute hospital admissions, which are very distressing for patients and families.
- Massive hemorrhages usually are fatal quickly; the main goal is to treat the patient's anxiety and help family members and staff to cope during the event. Expect major stress and additional bereavement needs.

### Unproductive Cough

- Unproductive coughs keep patients and family members awake at night and interfere with rest.
- Carefully evaluate for chronic aspiration and teach aspiration precautions.
- Avoid ACE inhibitors such as captopril (Capoten), treat bronchitis, consider tapping of pleural effusions or a trial of bronchodilators.[58]
- Minimize use of volume expanders like blood transfusions or IV saline.
- Increase the dose of opioids or try opioid cough suppressants, benzonate perles (Tessalon), nebulized saline or lidocaine, or sedatives, if needed.
- To dry up secretions, add an anticholinergic such as glycopyrrolate (Robinul) or transdermal scopolamine (Transderm Scop).

### Malodorous Wounds, Stomas, Tumors

- Patients are intensely embarrassed by malodorous wounds and stomas.
- Debride wounds when necessary.
- Use metronidazole gel or oral metronidazole 250 mg three times a day or other treatments like chloramphenicol to reduce anaerobes.
- Apply half-strength Dakens solution to bandages, or try activated charcoal pads.
- Involve an enterostomal therapist to provide patient and family education concerning appliances and portable deodorizing machines; avoid use of household sprays.

### Acute Confusional or Delusional States

- Confusion can cause wandering and increased anxiety and insomnia.
- Paranoid states cause intense caregiver distress due to the patient's accusations of cruel treatment, murder conspiracies, etc.
- Thoroughly investigate medical causes, including medication side effects, and treat aggressively, as appropriate.
- If no reversible cause can be found, try sedation with haloperidol or chlorpromazine in younger patients or risperidone or olanzapine in the elderly.
- Supply families with parenteral sedatives like haloperidol for SC use if oral medications are refused or ineffective.
- Add haloperidol (and midazolam if necessary) to SC infusions of opioids to prevent recurrent crises.
- Until the crisis passes, physicians and other members of the team should visit more often, continuous care may be needed in the home (see "Levels of Care" on page 62), or the patient may need to be admitted for inpatient treatment.

# Common Ethical Issues in the Home Care Setting

Several ethical issues commonly occur in the home setting, including the following have been described by Doyle.[50] For more information, see *UNIPAC Six: Ethical and Legal Decision Making When Caring for the Terminally Ill.*

- **Confidentiality, autonomy, and cultural expectations.** Patients have a right to know their diagnosis, prognosis, and treatment options regardless of the family's wishes to withhold such information. It is also important to recognize that some patients do not want to hear such information and should not be forced to listen to it. In some cases, sharing bad news contradicts the norms and expectations of specific cultural groups whose values should be honored. Resolving competing information-related needs can be difficult, particularly in hospice/palliative care settings where the patient *and* family are the unit of care. Without the patient's permission, physicians should not share confidential information with others, including family members, team members, or the patient's minister, rabbi, or spiritual leader. See UNIPACs Five and Six.

- **Safety versus independence.** Family members and healthcare professionals may be more concerned about a patient's safety than the patient, who may be more interested in maintaining a sense of independence. Concerns about safety can result in the patient's being confined to bed or transferred to a nursing facility before the patient is ready to do so. In some cases, interventions allow patients to remain at home longer, e.g., rearranging the home setting to reduce safety hazards, scheduling additional visits from hospice/palliative team members, volunteers, neighbors, and church members, and involving physical and occupational therapists in the patient's care. Every effort should be made to respect the patient's wishes and to prevent crises that precipitate unwanted transfers to other care settings.

- **Treating the patient for the family's sake.** Treating symptoms that are not distressing for the patient but contribute to the family's suffering can be ethically complex, e.g., treating a patient's death rattle with hyoscyamine or glycopyrrolate to reduce secretions so that the noise does not distress the family, even though the treatment dries the patient's mouth, or continuing artificial nutrition in a terminally ill cancer patient long enough to educate family members about the benefits and burdens of artificial nutrition. See UNIPAC Six.

- **Sedating the patient for the family's sake.** It is ethically acceptable to offer sedation to a patient whose distressing symptoms cannot be controlled even with expert palliative care.[59,60] However, patients should not be sedated against their will regardless of the family's wishes. Instead, interventions should be initiated to relieve the suffering of the patient and family. The patient may need aggressive interventions to alleviate physical, psychological, or spiritual pain. The family should receive increased emotional support and periodic relief from caregiving responsibilities, whenever possible. See UNIPACs Two, Three, Four, and Six.

## Hospice/Palliative Care for Vulnerable Patients in Institutional and Other Settings

Care of the dying is challenging in the best of circumstances. When the patient is a child in an institutional setting or in foster care, or an adult inmate in a prison, or a resident of a nursing home, it can be more difficult. Several inspiring programs, however, have demonstrated the possibility of success.

In the past 15 years the number of people dying in prison has risen sharply. In 1987 there were 1,400 deaths in American prisons, and by 1998 that number reached over 3,200.[61] From 1990 to 1997 the number of prisoners over the age of 55 doubled to reach nearly 50,000.[62] The large majority of these prisoners do not have access to palliative care, but over 26 facilities have started hospice programs for prisoners.[63] These programs often allow increased visitation, movement of prisoners within the prison, occasional amenities, and eventually procedures for dispensing adequate amounts of pain medication.[64] Fellow prisoners are sometimes trained to function as a surrogate family for lonely dying patients.[65]

The care of hospice patients in nursing homes entails other challenges. Nearly one in five older Americans dies in a nursing home, and many more die in hospitals after being institutionalized.[66] There is ample evidence that the care of dying patients in nursing homes is hampered by poor symptom management[67] and inadequate psychosocial support. Research suggests, however, that hospice enrollment is associated with higher-quality symptom assessment and management and with lower rates of hospitalization.[68,69] In 1997 the Office of the Inspector General issued a controversial report suggesting that 16% of nursing home patients admitted to hospice programs did not qualify for the Medicare Hospice Benefit.[70] This action caused many hospices to restrict admission of nursing home patients to those near death. There is continued concern about the quality of nursing home care, particularly for the most frail and vulnerable.[71] Hospice and palliative care can be part of that answer.[72]

For information on pediatric hospice/palliative care, see *UNIPAC Eight: The Hospice/Palliative Medicine Approach to Caring for Pediatric Patients.*

*A decent society cares for its most vulnerable members, including children and the elderly. As our society ages, it may be necessary to increase our spending to honor that commitment. What we need to be sure of is that we get our money's worth.*

—MARCIA ANGELL, MD[73]

*The United States is the only advanced industrial society in the world where a patient's ability to pay determines access to health care.*

—VOGELZANG, ET. AL[74]

## Costs of End-of-Life Care

Recommendations to improve end-of-life care include regulatory changes in U.S. health care financing.[75] Medical care at the end of life consumes 10% to 12% of the total health care budget and 28% of the Medicare budget.[76] Because the population is aging and millions of baby boomers are approaching retirement age, cost pressures are escalating and policy makers are concentrating on reducing healthcare costs associated with end-of-life care.[77] Cost-reduction efforts are focusing on Medicare for several reasons, including the following:[78]

- Medicare accounts for about 20% of personal healthcare expenditures in the United States and 11% of the United States federal budget.[79,80]
- 28% of all Medicare costs are spent on care during the last year of life; with almost 50% of these costs expended during the last 2 months of life[37]
- Since 1969, the rate of Medicare inflation has outstripped the consumer price index on an annual basis, averaging about 10% per beneficiary per year.
- The number of beneficiaries has grown steadily and will grow more rapidly as the baby boomers reach retirement age.
- Medicare Part A's trust fund, which pays for hospital, hospice, skilled-nursing, and home health care, is being depleted.
- Costs associated with Medicare Part B, which pays for physician services and outpatient care, are increasing rapidly.

- Improper reimbursement due to fraud and abuse is being blamed for up to 12% of Medicare expenditures.

Some experts believe that Medicare inflation is being driven by rapid growth in the components of the Medicare system that are less regulated than hospitals, for example, skilled nursing facilities, hospice care, home health care, and outpatient services.[56] The same experts acknowledge that, without adequate research, it is difficult to tell if increased growth in these areas represents the use of more appropriate forms of care or other factors, such as increasing numbers of for-profit nursing facilities, hospice programs, and home health care agencies. In any case, hospice care accounts for only about 1% of Medicare spending and about one-tenth of 1% of Medicaid spending.[81]

## Impact of Hospice/Palliative Care on Healthcare Costs

More than a dozen studies have measured the impact of hospice care on healthcare costs. Although hospice care appears to be cost effective, estimates of the exact amount of savings vary widely. A study by Lewin-VHI, commissioned by the NHPCO, compared the costs of hospice care with conventional care and concluded that Medicare saves $1.52 for every $1.00 spent on hospice care.[82] Emanuel examined several recent studies and concluded that hospice care and the use of advance directives can save 10% to 17% of healthcare costs during the last 6 months of life, with savings increasing to between 25% and 40% in the last month, due primarily to reductions in hospital care.[77] According to Emanuel, a definitive study of costs has not yet been published, and methodological problems interfere with comparisons among current studies. Although cost savings associated with hospice care may not be as high throughout the entire illness trajectory as initially anticipated, Emanuel suggests that the use of hospice care and advance directives should be encouraged.

Despite its emphasis on palliative rather than curative interventions, hospice care is intensive and sometimes involves considerable expense for the following reasons:

- The goal of keeping patients at home for as long possible may require intensive support from the entire interdisciplinary team and frequent home visits by physicians, home health aides, homemakers, nurses, social workers, counselors, and chaplains.
- Comprehensive hospice/palliative care provides complex interventions for alleviating the physical, psychological, social, and spiritual components of suffering. Needed interventions often require the skills of an entire interdisciplinary team of healthcare professionals, including physicians, nurses, social workers, and chaplains.
- Interventions to palliate difficult symptoms may require large quantities of expensive medications and perhaps even radiation therapy, chemotherapy, or surgery.

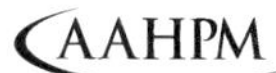

# Medicare Hospice Benefit

Medicare was designed to provide comprehensive medical care for older Americans. The benefit is divided into two sections:

- Part A provides hospital insurance.
- Part B provides voluntary supplementary medical insurance.

In 1982, the Tax Equity and Fiscal Responsibility Act (TEFRA) established the Medicare Hospice Benefit, which was first offered in 1983. The Medicare Hospice Benefit, an additional benefit of Medicare Part A, covers comprehensive end-of-life care primarily for elderly, terminally ill patients in the United States.

Medicare Part A is an 80/20 benefit: Medicare reimburses for 80% of the costs associated with care and patients are responsible for the other 20%. However, the Medicare Hospice Benefit is essentially a 100% benefit; all services are provided without cost to the beneficiary, as long as the services are covered by Medicare and are included in the patient's plan of care for palliative treatment of a terminal condition. Medicare-certified hospice programs can charge patients a 5% co-pay for respite care and for drugs needed to manage the terminal illness.

Medicare-eligible patients receiving services from Medicare-certified hospice programs do not receive bills from the hospice program for Medicare-covered hospice services; however, they are financially responsible for services not included in their individual plan of care or covered by the Medicare Hospice Benefit. Patients continue to be responsible for the usual 20% co-pay for visits to their attending physician.

To receive the hospice benefit, patients waive traditional Medicare Part A and elect the Medicare Hospice Benefit (MHB), which covers all healthcare services related to the terminal diagnosis, including prescription medications. After choosing the hospice benefit, patients are still covered by traditional Medicare Part A for care unrelated to the terminal illness. For example, a terminally ill patient elects the hospice benefit, is subsequently hit by a car, and needs care for a broken leg. The MHB continues to provide coverage for costs related to the person's terminal illness, but traditional Medicare Part A assumes coverage of care related to the broken leg.

The Medicare Hospice Benefit has improved end-of-life care for thousands of people in the United States by supporting comprehensive interventions to relieve physical, emotional, social, and spiritual pain. In the early 1990s, 20% of terminally ill patients chose the Medicare Hospice Benefit.[83] In 2000, approximately one of every four people who died in the United States from all causes received hospice care. Factors contributing to continuing low usage of the hospice benefit include the following:

- Widespread cultural denial and fear of death (see UNIPAC Two)
- Lack of awareness of the benefit on the part of the public and healthcare professionals (75% of Americans do not realize that hospice care can be provided in the home and 90% do not understand that hospice care can be fully covered through Medicare[37])
- Patient or family reluctance to make the transition from curative to palliative care[84]
- Physicians' concerns about accurately predicting prognosis, including overestimating a patient's survival[88] (see "Certification of Terminal Illness" on page 56)
- Concerns about the definition of palliative treatment and the costs associated with aggressive palliative interventions

## Eligibility Criteria for the Medicare Hospice Benefit

Table 18 lists eligibility criteria for the Medicare Hospice Benefit.

**Table 18: Eligibility Criteria for the Medicare Hospice Benefit**

**Patient Is Eligible for Medicare Part A**

- Usually anyone is eligible who is 65 years of age or older or receives Medicare disability payments.

**Patient Has a Terminal Condition**

- Two physicians must sign a statement certifying that the patient's medical prognosis suggests a life expectancy of 6 months or less, based on the physician's or medical director's clinical judgment regarding the normal course of the individual's illness.[86] One of the physicians must be the hospice medical director or the hospice team physician; the other is the patient's attending physician.
- When the hospice medical director also serves as the patient's attending physician, only the signature of the medical director is required.

**Patient Chooses Hospice Care—Informed Consent**

- The patient chooses hospice care and signs a MHB election form.

**Care Is Provided by a Medicare-certified Hospice Program**

- All care for the terminal condition is provided by a Medicare-certified hospice program

## Benefit Periods

In 1997, the federal Budget Reconciliation Bill contained provisions that altered several aspects of the Medicare Hospice Benefit, including benefit periods. The Reconciliation Bill restructured the periods, which now consist of two 90-day periods followed by an unlimited number of 60-day periods. Before one benefit period ends and the next one begins, the hospice medical director or physician member of the interdisciplinary team is responsible for reevaluating the patient and recertifying that the patient is terminally ill with a prognosis that suggests a life expectancy of 6 months or less if the disease runs it normal course. Without certification and recertification, patients are not eligible for continued hospice care under the Medicare Hospice Benefit.

Patients may revoke the hospice benefit at any time by signing a revocation form; however, revocation results in the loss of all remaining days in that benefit period. If patients decide to resume the hospice benefit, they must be reevaluated and recertified by two physicians who certify a life expectancy of 6 months or less if the disease runs its normal course. If certified as terminally ill, the patient signs a hospice election form and is placed in the next benefit period. When patients revoke the hospice benefit, traditional Medicare is immediately available.

## Certification of Terminal Illness

One primary responsibility of a hospice medical director is certifying a patient's life expectancy as 6 months or less. Because life expectancy is difficult to predict, particularly for noncancer diseases, physicians may be reluctant to certify patients as terminally ill until very late in the illness, depriving patients and families of much needed symptom control and emotional support until the last few weeks of the patient's life. Predicting prognosis is particularly difficult in the following situations:

- Patients with diseases such as chronic heart failure, pulmonary disease, and neurological conditions
- Patients with diseases such as AIDS, who may experience periodic bouts of serious illness followed by periods of remission when treated aggressively
- Patients who live longer than expected due to effective symptom control and emotional and spiritual support

Physicians' concerns about accurate prognostication have been exacerbated by the U.S. Inspector General's Office, which investigates fraud and abuse in the Medicare program. The Office has focused its investigations on rapidly growing sectors of the healthcare industry, e.g., home health agencies, skilled nursing facilities, suppliers of durable medical equipment, and hospice programs. In the hospice sector, the Office is concerned about patients not meeting eligibility requirements for the Medicare Hospice Benefit, in particular the requirement that patients have a prognosis of 6 months or less if the disease runs its normal course. The Benefits Improvement and Protection Act of 2000 (BIPA) clarified the benefit's definition of *terminally ill*. The new definition states that the determination of a 6-month-or-less prognosis is to be "based on the physician's or medical director's judgment regarding the normal course of the individual's illness."[86]

## Criteria for Predicting Prognosis for Noncancer Diagnoses

In 2000, 57% of hospice patients were diagnosed with cancer upon admission.[37] The top five noncancer diagnoses were end-stage heart disease (10%), dementia (6%), lung disease (6%), end-stage kidney disease (3%), and end-stage liver disease (2%). To help physicians to determine a patient's appropriateness for hospice care, the NHPCO developed guidelines for identifying patients with noncancer illnesses who are likely to have a life expectancy of 6 months or less if the illness were to run its normal course.[87] The *Medical Guidelines for Determining Prognosis in Selected Non-Cancer Diseases* also may be useful for determining patient eligibility for the Medicare or Medicaid Hospice Benefit.[87] The *Guidelines* include general information about prognosis and specific guidelines for determining the prognosis of patients with selected noncancer diseases. Whenever possible, the *Guidelines* were based on scientific studies of mortality in noncancer disease, but they remain a consensus document that is not yet evidence based. The authors of the guidelines recognize the need for ongoing research to establish the criteria's accuracy and predictive validity.[88] See Table 19 for a summary of the *Guidelines*.

Medicare's regional fiscal intermediaries have adopted the guidelines as parameters for determining Medicare coverage for specific noncancer diagnoses. In some cases, the intermediaries altered the guidelines and incorporated them in local medical review policies for determining patient eligibility for Medicare coverage and, subsequently, for program reimbursement for care. It remains to be seen how BIPA's clarification of the definition will affect these policies.

Policies for each diagnosis allow individual consideration of patients not meeting specific criteria, who may be hospice appropriate due to other comorbidities or rapid decline. In such cases, comorbidities and/or rapid decline should be documented aggressively for patients who appear to be terminally ill but do not fit *Guidelines* criteria. Patients who stabilize will need to be discharged by the end of the first or second 90-day benefit period. Ongoing research is likely to contribute to further negotiations between hospice providers and the Centers for Medicare and Medicaid Services (formerly HCFA) for years to come.[89]

## Services Covered

Regardless of care setting, Medicare-certified hospice programs are required to provide certain services, as long as the services are required to palliate the symptoms of a termi-

## Table 19: Summary of the NHO Guidelines for Determining Prognosis

**General:** A life-limiting condition with evidence of either disease progression and/or impaired nutritional status indicated by involuntary weight loss ≥10% of body weight in past 6 months. Serum albumin ≤2.5 is a helpful but not necessary factor. The goal of treatment is relief of symptoms, not cure.

| Disease | Primary Factors | Secondary Factors |
|---|---|---|
| **Heart disease** | ■ Symptoms of recurrent heart failure or angina at rest, discomfort with any activity (NYHA Class IV)<br>■ Patient already optimally treated with diuretics and vasodilators, i.e., ACE inhibitors | ■ Ejection fraction ≤20%<br>■ Symptomatic arrhythmias<br>■ History of cardiac arrest and CPR<br>■ Unexplained syncope<br>■ Embolic CVA of cardiac origin<br>■ HIV disease |
| **Pulmonary disease** | ■ Disabling dyspnea at rest<br>■ Progressive pulmonary disease, e.g., increasing ER visits or hospitalizations for pulmonary infections and/or respiratory failure<br>■ Hypoxemia at rest on supplemental $O_2$<br>$pO_2 \leq 55$ mm Hg on supplemental $O_2$<br>$O_2$ sat ≤ 88% on supplemental $O_2$<br>*or*<br>Hypercapnia: $pCO_2 \geq 50$ mm HG | ■ $FEV_1$ after bronchodilator < 30% of predicted<br>■ Decreased $FEV_1$ on serial testing > 40 mL per year<br>■ Unintentional weight loss > 10% of body weight in 6 months<br>■ Resting tachycardia > 100/min in patient with severe chronic COPD<br>■ Documented cor pulmonale or right heart failure due to advanced pulmonary disease |
| **Dementia** | ■ Severity of dementia ≥ FAST Stage 7-C:<br>Unable to walk, dress, or bathe without assistance<br>Urinary and fecal incontinence<br>Unable to speak more than six different intelligible words per day<br>■ Severe comorbid condition within past 6 months:<br>Aspiration pneumonia<br>Pyelonephritis<br>Septicemia<br>Multiple, progressive stage 3 to 4 decubiti<br>Fever after antibiotics<br>■ Unable to maintain fluid/caloric intake to sustain life | |

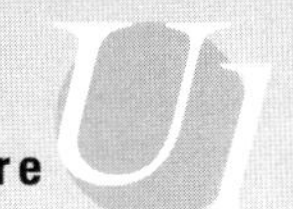

| Disease | Primary Factors | Secondary Factors |
|---|---|---|
| | ■ If feeding tube in place:<br>Wt. loss > 10% in 6 months<br>serum albumin <2.5 g/dl | |
| **HIV disease** (*Note:* Criteria established prior to the availability of highly effective antiretroviral therapy.) | ■ CD4+ < 25 cells/μL<br>*or*<br>Viral load ≥ 100,000 copies/mL<br>■ Karnovsky ≥ 50%<br>■ One of the following:<br>CNS lymphoma<br>Progressive multifocal leukoencephalopathy<br>Advanced dementia<br>Cryptosporidiosis<br>Wasting > 33%<br>Toxoplasmosis<br>Visceral KS, no Rx<br>MAC bacteremia, no Rx<br>Renal failure, no dialysis | ■ Forgoing antiretroviral and prophylactic drug Rx<br>■ Chronic, persistent diarrhea for 1 year<br>■ Albumin < 2.5 g/dL<br>■ Age > 50 yr<br>■ CHF, NYHA Class IV<br>■ Active substance abuse<br>*Note:* A Karnovsky performance score ≤50% indicates the patient requires considerable assistance and frequent medical care. |
| **Liver disease** | ■ End-stage cirrhosis; not a candidate for liver transplant<br>■ PT > 5 sec over control or INR > 1.5 *and* serum albumin < 2.5 g/dL<br>■ At least one of the following:<br>Ascites despite treatment<br>Spontaneous peritonitis<br>Hepatorenal syndrome<br>Hepatic encephalopathy despite treatment<br>Recurrent variceal bleed | ■ Progressive malnutrition<br>■ Muscle wasting<br>■ Continued alcoholism<br>■ Primary liver cancer<br>■ Positive HBsAg |
| **Renal disease** | ■ Chronic renal failure; coming off or not a candidate for dialysis<br>■ Creatinine clearance < 10 cc/min (for diabetics < 15 cc/min) *and* serum creatinine > 8.0 mg/dL (for diabetics > 6.0 mg/dl)<br>■ Signs and symptoms associated with renal failure<br>Uremia: nausea, pruritus, confusion, or restlessness<br>Oliguria: output < 400 cc/24 h<br>Intractable hyperkalemia: serum K >7.0<br>Uremic pericarditis<br>Hepatorenal syndrome<br>Intractable fluid overload | ■ Mechanical ventilation<br>■ Malignancy, other organ system<br>■ Chronic lung disease<br>■ Advanced cardiac or liver disease<br>■ Sepsis<br>■ Immunosuppression/HIV<br>■ Cachexia or albumin < 3.5 g/dL<br>■ Age > 75 yr<br>■ Platelets < 25,000<br>■ GI bleed<br>■ Disseminated intravascular coagulation |

(*Continued*)

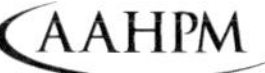

| | | |
|---|---|---|
| **Stroke and coma** | *Acute phase following CVA:*<br>■ Coma or persistent vegetative state > 3 days<br>■ Any four of the following on day 3 of coma:<br>Abnormal brain stem response<br>Absent verbal response<br>Absent withdrawal to pain<br>Serum creatine > 1.5 mg/dL<br>■ Unable to maintain fluid/caloric intake to sustain life<br>*Chronic phase of CVA*:<br>■ Any one of the following:<br>Age > 70 yr<br>Poststroke dementia: FAST score > 7<br>Karnovsky ≤ 50%<br>Poor nutritional status; see above | ■ Aspiration pneumonia<br>■ Upper urinary tract infection e.g., pyelonephritis<br>■ Sepsis<br>■ Progressive refractory stage 3 to 4 decubiti<br>■ Fever after antibiotics<br>*Note:* A Karnovsky score ≤ 50% indicates the patient requires considerable assistance and frequent medical care. |
| **Amyotrophic Lateral Sclerosis (ALS)** | ■ Critically impaired ventilatory capacity indicated by:<br>Vital capacity < 30% of predicted<br>Significant dyspnea at rest<br>Requires $O_2$ at rest<br>Declines intubation, tracheostomy, mechanical ventilation<br>*or*<br>■ Rapid progression and critical nutritional impairment indicated by:<br>Oral intake of nutrients or fluids insufficient to sustain life<br>Continued weight loss<br>Dehydration or hypovolemia<br>*or*<br>■ Rapid progression and life-threatening complications such as:<br>Aspiration pneumonia<br>Upper urinary infection, i.e., pyelonephritis<br>Sepsis<br>Multiple, progressive stage 3 to 4 decubiti<br>Fever recurrent after antibiotics | |

Summarized with permission from the NHPCO's *Medical Guidelines for Determining Prognosis in Selected Non-Cancer Diseases*, 2nd ed. 

**Table 20: Required Services Covered by the Medicare Hospice Benefit**

All the following services are required and covered if they are needed to palliate the symptoms of a terminal diagnosis and are included in the patient's plan of care:

- Medicines and biologicals
- Durable medical equipment (hospital bed, walker, oxygen concentrator, etc.)
- Medical supplies
- Laboratory services
- X-ray and radiation therapy
- Emergency services
- Ambulance and transport services
- Short-term inpatient stays in a hospice facility, hospital, or skilled care facility for management of acute symptoms
- Short-term continuous nursing care in the home for crisis care of acute symptoms that can be managed at home with extra support from the hospice team
- Five-day inpatient respite periods when caretakers require a break from caregiving responsibilities
- Bereavement support and counseling services
- Use of an interdisciplinary team
  Medical supervision
  Physician services
  Individual case management and coordination of care by a registered nurse
  Intermittent nursing visits
  Social work services
  Pastoral counseling and spiritual support provided or coordinated by a hospice chaplain
  Home health aide and homemaker services
  Volunteer services
  Dietary counseling and physical, occupational, speech, and respiratory therapy services as appropriate

nal diagnosis and are included in the patient's plan of care (see Table 20). Other Medicare services may also be covered if they are included in the patient's plan of care.

See Table 21 for a comparison of the services covered by the Medicare Hospice Benefit and the Medicare Home Health Benefit.

**Table 21: Comparison of the Medicare Hospice Benefit and the Medicare Home Care Benefit**

| Service | Medicare Hospice | Medicare Home Health |
|---|---|---|
| 100% coverage of medications to control pain and other symptoms related to the terminal illness (hospice programs can charge a 5% co-payment) | Yes | No |
| 100% coverage of durable medical equipment and medical supplies without a deductible or co-payment | Yes | No |
| Homemakers and home health aides | Yes | Yes, if short term |
| Inpatient respite care (hospice programs can charge a 5% co-payment) | Yes | No |
| Inpatient care with no deductible | Yes | No |
| Continuous RN care in the home during periods of medical crisis | Yes | No |
| Counseling in the home for patient and family | Yes | Limited |
| Bereavement support | Yes | No |
| Trained volunteers | Yes | No |
| Professional management and supervision of care in all settings, including inpatient | Yes | No |
| Ongoing pastoral counseling and spiritual support for patients and family | Yes | No |
| Payment of consulting physician fees at 100% | Yes | No |
| Physician, nurse, social worker, and counselor on-call availability 24 hours a day, 7 days a week | Yes | No |
| Family supportive care | Yes | No |
| Patient must be homebound | No | Yes |

## Levels of Care

In 2000, the Medicare hospice benefit provided per diem reimbursement based on the four levels of care described in Table 22:

- Routine home care: about $110
- Continuous home care: about $644

## Table 22: Medicare Hospice Levels of Care

**Routine Home Care**

For routine home care provided in the patient's place of residence, whether a private home, a nursing facility, or prison.[37,90] The benefit does not cover the cost of a patient's room and board in a nursing home. The hospice is reimbursed at the routine home care rate for each day that the patient is enrolled in the hospice program and is not receiving another level of care. The same rate is paid for each day of routine home care regardless of the volume or intensity of services provided on a given day. The home care rate is adjusted for locale. The routine home care rate also is paid when:

- Patients are in the hospital for conditions unrelated to the terminal illness
- Patients are in a hospital that does not contract with the hospice
- Patients are receiving outpatient services in the hospital
- The day the patient is discharged alive from inpatient or respite care

**Continuous Home Care**

For crisis management of acute symptoms to maintain the patient at home. Continuous care:

- Requires predominantly intensive nursing care to achieve palliation or management of acute symptoms
- Must be provided for a minimum of 8 hours during each 24-hour day, with each day beginning at midnight
- Does not have to be continuous; staff can be assigned for a 4-hour period in the morning and a 4-hour period at night, but 51% of the care provided during each period must require the services of licensed nurses. The remainder may be provided by home health aides.
- Requires careful hour-by-hour documentation of the patient's physical condition, services provided, and personnel needed
- Is billed by the hour if intensive services are provided for more than 8 hours, but less than 24 hours. If fewer than 8 hours of intensive services are required, the days are reimbursed at the routine home care rate.

**General Inpatient Care**

For control of acute pain or other symptoms that cannot be adequately managed in the patient's home.

- Inpatient acute care is short-term care provided by a contracted hospice facility, hospital, or skilled nursing facility.
- Inpatient acute care may be needed for pain and symptom management, support during the active phase of dying, and management of complicated psychosocial issues. Custodial care only does not qualify the patient for general inpatient care.
- The hospice program continues to serve as the professional manager of the patient regardless of inpatient setting, and all services provided must conform with the patient's Plan of Care.

(*Continued*)

- The hospice program is reimbursed at the general inpatient care rate for every day that the patient is in a contracted facility and is receiving the general inpatient level of care, including the day of admission.
- If the patient is discharged alive, the program is reimbursed at the home care rate for the day of discharge. If the patient dies while in the inpatient facility, the program is reimbursed at the inpatient rate for the day of discharge

**Respite Care**
For patients whose caregivers need relief:

- Respite care is reimbursed for no more than 5 days at a time in a contracted hospice facility, hospital, skilled nursing facility, or intermediate care facility.
- Reimbursement for the sixth and subsequent days is at the home care rate.
- The hospice program continues to provide professional management of the patient's care and the services provided must conform with the patient's Plan of Care.
- Although the number of respite stays is not limited to a specific number, documentation should clearly indicate why respite care is needed, particularly if it occurs frequently.
- The patient is liable for a 5% co-payment if the hospice program chooses to charge for it.

- General inpatient care: about $490
- Respite care: about $120

In 2000, 96% of hospice days of service were categorized as routine home care, 3% as general inpatient care, and less than one-half of 1% were for respite care and continuous care.[35] In 2001, the Centers for Medicare and Medicaid Services increased payment rates for hospice care services by 5%.

## Plan of Care

The Medicare Hospice Benefit requires an individualized Plan of Care for each patient–family unit. With input from the patient and family, members of the interdisciplinary team develop a comprehensive care plan designed to meet the patient's physical needs *and* the psychological, spiritual, and social needs of the patient and family. The hospice program is financially responsible for providing all services needed for palliation of a terminal diagnosis, as long as they are identified in a patient's Plan of Care and are covered by Medicare. Care plans identify the following:

- The patient's and family's problems
- The patient's and family's strengths and existing resources

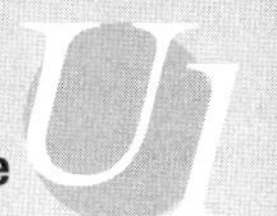

- Interventions needed to alleviate sources of physical, emotional, spiritual, and social distress related to the terminal illness

For more information about hospice interdisciplinary teams, see *UNIPAC Five: Caring for the Terminally Ill—Communication and the Physician's Role on the Interdisciplinary Team.* For additional information, see the NHPCO publication, A *Pathway for Patients and Families Facing Terminal Illness.*

## Hospice Program Reimbursement

The Centers for Medicare and Medicaid Services (CMA), (formerly the Health Care Financing Administration, (HCFA) sets national reimbursement rates for each of the four levels of care described in Table 22. The national rates are adjusted according to the wage index for each area of the country. Medicare contracts with regional fiscal intermediaries, who review submitted bills for accuracy and appropriateness. Medicare-certified hospice programs are reimbursed on a per diem basis according to each patient's level of care, regardless of the intensity of services provided on a specific day.

### Limits on Reimbursement

The Medicare Hospice Benefit includes two provisions that limit program reimbursement: a limit on inpatient care and an aggregate cap on overall program reimbursement.

**Limit on payment for inpatient care.** The Medicare Hospice Benefit encourages home-based care by limiting reimbursement for inpatient care. During each 12-month period beginning on November 1, a hospice program's aggregate number of inpatient days (for both general inpatient care and inpatient respite care) may not exceed 20% of the aggregate total number of days of hospice care provided for all Medicare beneficiaries during that same period.[91] If a hospice program exceeds the 20% limit on inpatient days, the program must refund excess reimbursement to Medicare. Reimbursement for inpatient days over the 20% limit is reduced to the routine home care rate.

Hospice inpatient care is intended for short-term management of acute symptoms or respite care. Because most patients remain at home (whether a private residence or a facility) throughout their illness or require only short-term inpatient stays, most hospice programs have no difficulty meeting the 20% limit. The exception tends to be hospice programs operating inpatient facilities without a large enough home care census to support the number of inpatient beds. Nationally, the inpatient care option may be underused; only 3% of the total number of days billed to the Medicare Hospice Benefit days are billed as inpatient days.[92]

**Aggregate cap on overall reimbursement.** Overall aggregate payments to hospice programs are subject to an annual cap amount that is calculated by the intermediary at the end of the hospice cap period. The cap period begins on November 1. The cap amount is calculated by multiplying the number of Medicare beneficiaries admitted to a hospice program during the cap period by an amount of money determined by statute. In 1990 the statutory amount was set at $6,500. The statutory amount is adjusted each year to reflect the percentage increase or decrease in the medical care expenditures of the Consumer Price Index for all urban consumers; by 1997, the amount increased to $13,974.

Each year the intermediary compares the program's aggregate cap amount with the amount of money Medicare paid to the program for hospice services furnished to Medicare beneficiaries during the cap period. Any payments in excess of the cap must be refunded by the hospice program. Payments are measured in terms of **all** payments made to hospice on behalf of **all** Medicare hospice beneficiaries receiving services during the cap year. The aggregate system was designed so that programs can provide expensive palliative interventions for the relatively few terminally ill patients who need them, for example, patients needing radiation therapy, chemotherapy, or surgical interventions. Because most patients do not require aggressive interventions and because the median patient survival after hospice enrollment was only 25 days,[37,93] most programs can provide comprehensive services for all patients without exceeding the aggregate cap.

### Length of Stay

In 2000, 33% of people served by hospice died in 7 days or less. Six percent died in 180 days or more. In 2000, the average length of stay was 48 days. Due to the high frequency of short stays, the median length of stay more accurately reflects the experience of a typical hospice patient. In 2000, the median length of stay was 25 days.[37]

## Medicaid Hospice Benefit

Medicaid is a state insurance program for citizens of any age who fall below the state's poverty income guidelines. In general, Medicaid covers acute care, long-term care, and custodial care in the patient's home. Many states offer a Medicaid Hospice Benefit, usually similar to the Medicare Hospice Benefit in terms of services, benefit periods, and recertification of terminal illness. However, some states set their own requirements. In many states, the Medicaid Hospice Benefit requirements are complex due to state Medicaid waivers and increased use of Medicaid HMOs. Physicians should inquire about state-specific requirements and benefits.

# Physician Reimbursement for Hospice/Palliative Medicine

## Medicare Hospice Benefit

Most physicians associated with hospice/palliative care programs serve in one of the following capacities:

- Attending physician not employed by the hospice program
- Hospice medical director or team physician employed by the hospice program
- Consulting physician

For information about the specific roles of physicians associated with hospice programs, see *UNIPAC Five: Caring for the Terminally Ill—Communication and the Physician's Role on the Interdisciplinary Team.*

### Attending Physician

Under the Medicare hospice benefit, the attending physician is the physician who has the most significant role in determining and delivering the patient's medical care. Patients choose their attending physician, who is responsible for their care. The attending physician must be a doctor of medicine or osteopathy and must be designated on the patient's Medicare hospice benefit election form as the attending physician. In most cases, the patient's usual attending physician continues to serve in that capacity after the patient is admitted for hospice/palliative care. The attending physician must designate a covering (stand-in) physician to care for the patient when the attending physician is on vacation or otherwise unavailable. The hospice medical director or a hospice-employed team physician can serve as an attending physician, if requested by the patient.

### Hospice Medical Director or Team Physician

Smaller hospice programs generally employ one physician who serves as a part-time or full-time medical director. Larger programs usually employ a full-time medical director and may also employ one or more team physicians, whose specific functions depend on the program's needs.

Medical directors and hospice team physicians contract directly with the hospice for reimbursement. Contracts are based on the number of hours that the physician is expected to work, the physician's training, experience, board certification in hospice and palliative medicine (the American Board of Hospice and Palliative Medicine certifies physicians in hospice/palliative medicine), and community reimbursement standards for similar positions. New provisions in the 1997 Budget Reconciliation Bill allow hospice programs to contract for physician services with independent contractor physicians or physician groups.

The medical director of a Medicare-certified hospice program or the director's designee (a hospice team physician) performs the following duties:

- Assumes overall responsibility for the medical component of the care plans for all hospice patients, including those who have elected the Medicare Hospice Benefit[92]
- Certifies and recertifies a patient's terminal illness
- Actively participates on the team to establish patient-specific plans of care
- Routinely reviews and updates the patients' plans of care to ensure that patients and families are receiving needed care and services
- Works collaboratively with the patient's attending physician

When a hospice medical director or team physician also serves as a patient's attending physician, the billing procedure for hospice-employed physicians is followed.

### Consulting Physicians

Other physicians providing patient services are classified as consulting physicians. Consulting physicians provide patient services documented as needed for palliation of a terminal diagnosis in the patient's Plan of Care. Consulting physicians contract with the hospice program and must bill the hospice program directly.

### Types of Services

The Medicare Hospice Benefit reimburses physicians for procedures and/or treatments necessary for the palliation of a patient's terminal illness. For purposes of reimbursement, the benefit classifies physician services as administrative or patient care. When physicians provide services for Medicare hospice patients that are unrelated to the terminal illness, they bill regular Medicare. See Table 23 for descriptions of the categories of service.

## Physician Reimbursement Process

The reimbursement process for physicians associated with Medicare-certified hospice programs depends on the physician's employment status and the types of services rendered. See Table 24 for a description of the Medicare Hospice Benefit's reimbursement procedures for attending and consulting physician services.

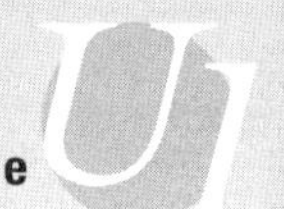

## Table 23: Types of Physician Services Reimbursed by the Medicare Hospice Benefit

**Administrative Services**

- *Physicians who are hospice employees.* Administrative services include attendance at team meetings, participation in the development of the patient's care plan, reviewing and updating the plan, supervising care and services, and establishing governing policies. These services are generally performed by the hospice medical director or the hospice team physician. Administrative services are included in the hospice program's per diem rate and are not billed separately. (This applies to the hospice program's medical director, staff physicians, or team physicians.)
- *Attending physicians who are not hospice employees.* Attending physicians who are not hospice employees do not bill the Medicare Hospice Benefit for administrative services or care plan oversight, but they may be able to bill traditional Medicare for such services.
- *Consulting physicians.* Consulting physicians do not bill for administrative services.

**Patient Care Services**

Patient care services include professional services provided by physicians who are employed by the hospice, by attending physicians who are not employed by the hospice, and by outside consultants who provide patient care when authorized by the hospice program. Examples professional patient care services include procedures performed by physicians that are designated by appropriate CPT codes. Professional services provided by physicians employed by the hospice or by consulting physicians are the only services for which the hospice program bills Medicare A, in addition to the per diem. Attending physicians who are not hospice employees continue to bill Medicare Part B directly for professional services.

Patient care services provided by physicians often include two components, a professional component and a technical component. For example, x-ray and laboratory services can include a professional component, e.g., reading the x-ray or interpreting the lab results, and a technical component, e.g., taking the x-ray or drawing blood. The technical component can be performed by a physician, but often is performed by other healthcare professionals. The technical component of a patient care service is included in the hospice program's per diem rate. To receive reimbursement for the technical component, hospice-employed physicians, attending physicians not employed by the hospice, and consulting physicians should negotiate a contractual rate directly with the hospice program.

- *Physicians who are hospice employees.* Physicians who are hospice employees (paid or volunteer) bill the hospice program directly for professional services. The hospice program bills Medicare Part A, which reimburses the program at the lesser of the actual charge or 100% of the Medicare reasonable charge for services. Payment is in addition to the per deim, but is subject to the cap. The program reimburses the physician at an agreed-upon rate.
- *Attending physicians who are not hospice employees.* Attending physicians who are not employees of the hospice program continue to bill Medicare Part B for professional services—home, office, inpatient, or nursing home visits—just as they would for nonhospice patients. Payment for services is made directly to the physician at 80% of the Medicare reasonable charge. Hospice patients are responsible for the usual Medicare co-pay. Attending physicians can bill for care plan oversight for hospice patients if they are the

(*Continued*)

designated attending physician, have signed the patient's care plan, and meet documentation guidelines and other regulations.[94]

- *Consulting physicians.* Consulting physicians bill the hospice directly for professional services. The hospice program bills Medicare Part A, which reimburses the program at the lesser of the actual charge or 100% of the Medicare reasonable charge for services. The hospice program reimburses the consultant physician at an agreed-upon rate.

Table 25 provides a summary of the billing procedures for services provided by physicians associated with hospice programs. In states offering a Medicaid hospice benefit, the process for reimbursement is similar to that used by Medicare. When billing for care provided to hospice patients or for palliative medicine consultations, physicians should use appropriate CPT codes.

## Table 24: Reimbursement Procedure Guidelines for Physician Services

**Hospice Physician: Hospice Program Employee or Volunteer**

- The hospice physician bills the hospice program for professional, administrative, and technical services.
- The program bills Medicare Part A for the physician's professional services.
- Medicare Part A reimburses the program for the physician's professional services at 100% of the Medicare allowed rate for that area; the hospice physician's services are included in the program's aggregate cap amount.
- The program reimburses the physician for professional, administrative, and technical services at a rate agreed upon in the program's contract with the physician.
- When the hospice physician is also the attending physician, the program reimburses for administrative and technical services out of its per diem payment at a rate agreed upon in the program's contract with the physician.

**Attending Physician: Not a Hospice Program Employee or Volunteer**

- The program notifies the Medicare Part B carrier that the physician has been designated as the hospice patient's attending physician.
- The attending physician bills Medicare Part B directly only for professional services.
- The intermediary reimburses the attending physician directly at 80% of the Medicare allowed rate; the patient's regular Medicare co-pay still applies.
- The entire reimbursement process is separate from the hospice program's per diem reimbursement; the physician's reimbursement for professional services is not counted against the program's aggregate cap.
- Technical services performed by a physician or other healthcare professional are covered in the program's per diem rate.

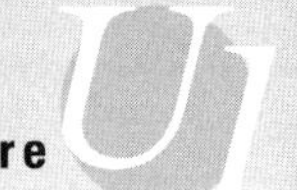

- The program reimburses the attending physician for technical services out of its per diem payment at an agreed-upon rate.

**Consulting Physician: Any Physician Who Provides Services but Is Not the Attending Physician**

- A consulting physician must have a contract with the hospice program.
- The need for medical treatment or services by a consulting physician must be documented in the patient's Plan of Care.
- The consulting physician must bill the hospice program directly for professional services; a consulting physician's bill is denied by the Medicare intermediary unless it is submitted through the hospice program.
- The program bills Medicare Part A for the consulting physician's professional services.
- The program receives reimbursement from Medicare Part A for 100% of the Medicare-allowed amount.
- The program reimburses the consulting physician at a rate agreed upon in the program's contract with the physician.
- Charges by a consulting physician are included in the program's aggregate cap.

**Table 25: Summary Chart for Physician Hospice Billing**

| Description of Service | Bill Medicare Part B | *Bill Hospice: Hospice Bills Intermediary and Reimburses Physician | *Bill Hospice: Covered under Hospice Benefit per Diem |
|---|---|---|---|
| **Attending Physician** | | | |
| Professional services | ✓ | | |
| **Covering (stand in) Physician** | | | |
| Professional services | ✓ | | |
| **Consulting Physician** | | | |
| Professional services | | ✓ | |
| **Hospice Medical Director (Volunteer or Paid)** | | | |
| Professional services | | ✓ | |
| Administrative services | | | ✓ |
| Technical services | | | ✓ |

*(Continued)*

| Description of Service | Bill Medicare Part B | *Bill Hospice: Hospice Bills Intermediary and Reimburses Physician | *Bill Hospice: Covered under Hospice Benefit per Diem |
|---|---|---|---|
| **X-rays** | | | |
| 1. Technical component | | | ✓ |
| 2. Professional services | | ✓ (consulting) | |
| **Radiation Therapy** | | | |
| 1. Technical component | | | ✓ |
| 2. Professional services | ✓ (attending) | ✓ (consulting) | |
| **Chemotherapy** | | | |
| 1. Technical component | | | ✓ |
| 2. Professional services | ✓ (attending) | ✓ (consulting) | |
| **Lab** | | | |
| 1. Technical component | | | ✓ |
| 2. Professional services | | ✓ (consulting) | |
| **Prescription Medications** | | | ✓ |

*The Medicare intermediary pays the hospice program an amount equivalent to 100% of allowable charges for physician services furnished under arrangements with the hospice program. The program reimburses the physician according to written agreements between the program and the covering physician and consulting physician. Physicians must bill the hospice program directly for services related to the terminal illness that are covered by the Medicare Hospice Benefit.

*Notes*

- The attending physician is the physician who has the most significant role in determining and delivering the patient's medical care. Bill Medicare Part B.
- The covering physician is the physician who sees the patient on behalf of the attending physician. Bill using the appropriate HCFA code.
- The consulting physician is the physician who provides direct patient care to a hospice patient for a condition related to the terminal illness. Bill the hospice program using the appropriate HCFA code.

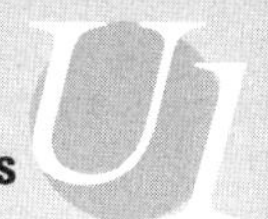

*Ethics, a process of interdisciplinary critical reflection, acts against a tendency to diverge systematically from what is right.*

—David J. Roy[94]

*For clinical ethics, the problems raised by suffering patients require us to face the fact that since these sick persons cannot enunciate their autonomy unaided, we must seek new ways by which their interests are to be truly represented within the community of their care.*

—Eric J. Cassel[13]

# Cultural and Religious Diversity

Roy suggests that modern societies can no longer expect universal agreement about what is right and good or wrong and bad.[96] The increasing diversity of cultural beliefs and religious traditions in modern pluralistic societies presents challenges to traditional methods of decision making. When patients, family members, physicians, and other healthcare professionals work together to make ethical decisions, they must pay careful attention to each participant's values, needs, and judgments.[97] By fully exploring the values and concerns of each participant, the process of corrective interplay usually results in the best possible decision for a specific situation. However, according to Roy, the process requires a shift from divergent to convergent methods of thinking. Only then can participants decide what must be done, what must be prohibited, and what can be tolerated.[96]

As patients and families make the transition from expecting a cure to preparing for death, they confront difficult issues, including the following:

- **The deeper meaning of changed treatment goals**. The switch from curative to palliative care means that the illness is incurable and life really is coming to an end.
- **Decisions about care settings.** The benefits and burdens of both home care and institutional care must be carefully considered, including the physical and psychological consequences for patients and family members. Burdens associated with home care include lack of sleep, the physical effort required when helping weakened patients to the bathroom or turning them every few hours, and lack of privacy. Benefits include an opportunity for increased sharing and closeness and a sense of continued involvement with family members.

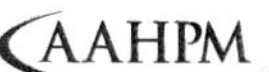

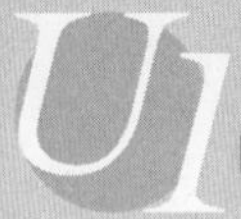



- **The devastating financial impact of terminal illness.** Prolonged terminal illnesses can easily consume a family's entire financial resources, especially families with little or no insurance and/or limited financial resources.
- **Existential loneliness.** Patients may lose their sense of hope, purpose, and meaning and believe that they are nothing but a burden to their families. They often need help reframing events and reestablishing a sense of hope and meaning.

## Autonomy and Serious Illness

The ethical principle of autonomy is valued so highly in hospice programs and in most Western cultures that all parties involved with care may have difficulty recognizing that a patient's ability to exercise autonomy can be compromised by profound illness. News of a life-threatening illness and the disease process itself can impair a patient's perceptions and ability to think clearly. Shock and stress may interfere with the ability of dying patients and their family members to clearly articulate their values and needs and to envision interventions that are in their best interests.[13,27]

Caught up in feelings of uncertainty, fear, and senselessness, terminally ill patients and family members often need assistance from compassionate healthcare professionals to help them to find meaning in what they are experiencing and to make decisions congruent with their values. Through a process of caring interaction and gentle probing, physicians can help patients and family members to:

- Articulate their beliefs, values, and goals
- Articulate their understanding of the situation and their associated fears and concerns
- Understand the diagnosis and its likely effects on daily life
- Understand the prognosis and its likely effects on future plans
- Understand symptoms and the benefits and burdens of various treatments
- Reassess their goals in light of new information
- Explore options and make decisions that reflect their values
- Reframe events and regain a sense of hope, purpose, and meaning

For more information on the ethical decision-making process and specific ethical issues related to hospice/palliative care, see *UNIPAC Six: Ethical and Legal Decision Making When Caring for the Terminally Ill.*

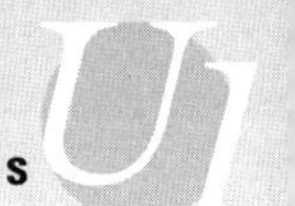

# Ethical Implications of an Organization's Policies

The NHPCO suggests that, due the extraordinary capacity for self-delusion demonstrated by individuals and organizations who may think that they are helping people when in fact they are doing just the opposite, organizations providing end-of-life care must develop policies that reflect the following:[98]

- Assessing the physical, emotional, spiritual, social, and financial needs of terminally ill patients and their families
- The ethical principles of beneficence, nonmaleficence, justice, autonomy, and nonabandonment
- Sensitivity to the beliefs, values, and coping strategies of people from diverse cultures

Ethical issues related to an organization's policies include:

- *Access to care*, e.g., denying care because patients have no insurance
- *Discontinuation of care*, e.g., discontinuing care because patients and/or family members have difficult personalities
- *Expensive palliative treatments*, e.g., withholding certain palliative interventions because they are considered to be too expensive

## Access to Care

The following characteristics describe Medicare beneficiaries enrolled in hospice programs. They suggest that hospice programs have been most successful at meeting the needs of white, elderly patients with cancer:[99]

- Mean age: 76.4 ± 9.0 years[93]
- 83% white[37]
- 60% cancer diagnosis[37]

Hospice programs have been less successful at meeting the needs of people with the following characteristics:[99,100]

- Less than 65 years of age
- A terminal disease or condition other than cancer
- Non-English speaking and/or non-Caucasian

- Ineligible for Medicare or Medicaid, no health insurance, few personal financial resources
- Live alone and/or are socially isolated
- Belong to a severely dysfunctional family
- Reside in unsafe environments, remote rural areas, prisons,[101] shelters, or other institutions
- No access to basic necessities: hot running water, heat, food, or income

### Policies That Limit Access to Care

Some hospice programs have established polices such as those described in Table 26, which may inadvertently serve as barriers to hospice care. Such policies are not supported by the Medicare Hospice Benefit or the NHPCO.

#### Table 26: Hospice Program Policies That May Limit Access to Care*

- **To be admitted, patients must have supportive families with a primary caretaker or sign a waiver promising to find one.** Fewer hospice programs are requiring a primary caretaker. In 1995, 60% of hospice programs did not require a primary caretaker and 27% reviewed patients on a case by case basis.[37] Many households cannot provide primary caregivers 24 hours a day because families are separated geographically, frail retired spouses are unable to provide care, and younger adult household members work and are absent for significant periods of time. Dying patients may also belong to dysfunctional family systems requiring extra support and creative solutions for challenging problems, e.g., mental disorders, drug abuse, weapons, attack dogs, etc.
- **Patients must discontinue certain therapies prior to admission.** Although much less common today, some programs do not accept patients who are receiving therapies that might be life prolonging, but also have palliative effects, e.g., chemotherapy, palliative radiation, or strontium 89 to control bone pain. In 1995, 53% of hospice programs accepted patients requiring high-tech therapies, and an additional 39% admitted such patients on a case by case basis.[37] As patients make the transition from curative to palliative care, they can benefit from symptom control and emotional and spiritual support services even when they are receiving aggressive palliative treatments. Some programs withhold aggressive palliative treatments that are considered too expensive.
- **Patients must agree to a DNR order.** Most programs do not require a DNR order for admission; by 1995, 76% of hospice programs admitted patients without DNR orders.[37] In some states requiring a DNR order is illegal. Misconceptions about the meaning of DNR orders and lack of knowledge about the results of CPR when used on frail, terminally ill patients may result in patient and family reluctance to withhold the procedure. Patients and families need information, guidance, symptom control, and emotional and spiritual support as they make the transition from curative to palliative care. Hospice programs are not required to provide futile treatment.

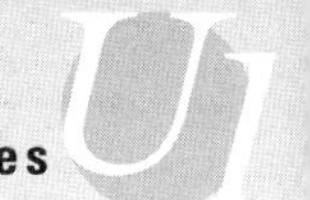

- **Patients must live in safe geographic locations.** Medicare-certified hospice programs cannot discriminate based on neighborhood. Due to real concerns about staff safety, some programs have developed creative strategies for providing services to patients who live in dangerous neighborhoods where gang-related activity, drug abuse, and weapons are common.
- **Patients must have a cancer diagnosis.** Although increasingly uncommon, some programs still accept only patients with cancer diagnoses. In 1995, 93% of programs admitted patients with a noncancer diagnosis.[37] Illnesses such as ALS, Alzheimer's, COPD, CHF, and AIDS have a less predictable prognosis than cancer, which contributes to concerns about complying with Medicare Hospice Benefit guidelines regarding length of life. Some physicians fear that they will be charged with fraud if they certify a noncancer patient as terminally ill and the patient lives longer than expected. Community physicians need more information about the NHPCO guidelines for determining eligibility for hospice care and the revised Medicare Hospice Benefit periods.
- **Patients must be of a certain age.** In 1995, 86% of programs accepted pediatric patients; however, only 1% of admitted patients were 17 or younger.[37] Pediatric patients often receive inadequate pain and symptom control in acute care settings and need specialized emotional and spiritual support during their terminal illness, as do their parents.
- **Patients must subscribe to specific religious traditions.** Some hospice programs were established by religious organizations whose chaplains were not familiar with other religious traditions and/or believed that only certain religious beliefs and practices were correct. Such programs may find it difficult to accommodate certain religious practices, especially in inpatient settings. For example, Muslims and Hindus often subscribe to strict bathing requirements; Hindus, Buddhists, Jews, and Muslims often observe strict dietary rules; and Hindus and Buddhists often place great emphasis on personal modesty. The alleviation of suffering requires observance of each patient's religious traditions. See *UNIPAC Two: Alleviating Psychological and Spiritual Pain in the Terminally Ill.*

*With the exception of age limits on Medicare eligibility, none of the above policies is supported by the Medicare Hospice Benefit or the NHPCO's standards of care.

To improve access for underserved populations, Brenner suggests that hospice/palliative care programs develop organizational policies that encourage the following:[99]

- Recruitment of staff reflecting racial and ethnic compositions of their service areas
- Training to help staff to work effectively with a wide range of cultural and religious beliefs and home settings
- Creation of outreach programs to provide services for all terminally ill patients as early as possible
- Coordination with other community programs, services, and institutions to provide services for the disenfranchised and to care for patients without basic financial and environmental necessities, e.g., income, heat, running water, food

## Discontinuation of Care

The following section is based on the NHPCO publication, *Discontinuation of Care: Ethical Principles.*[98] Discontinuation of care usually results from one of the following events:

- Withdrawal from the program
- Transfer to a different program
- Discharge from the program
- Revocation of the hospice benefit
- Nonrecertification of a terminal illness with a likely prognosis of 6 months or less

On some occasions, discontinuation of services can be avoided by:

- Ensuring adequate informed consent during the admission process, e.g., careful explanations of the goals of palliative care and the services provided by the hospice program
- Including patients and families in the process of developing the patient's Plan of Care

Because illness and stress interfere with a patient's or family's ability to hear and retain information, hospice programs should provide written explanations of the following:

- The goals of palliative treatments compared to curative treatments
- The services a Medicare-certified program is required to provide
- The services provided by this particular hospice program
- Inclusion of the patient and family when developing the patient's Plan of Care to ensure that interventions meet their needs
- The process of negotiating differences between the patient and family and the program
- Reasons for discontinuing hospice services and the consequences of each type of discontinuation
- Grievance procedures

When services are discontinued for any reason, the program should explain and document the entire process and continue all services until the discharge is completed.

### Withdrawal from the Hospice Program

Withdrawal is initiated by the patient or family. Patients may withdraw from a hospice program at any time for any reason.

### Transfer to a Different Hospice Program

Transfer to a different program is initiated by the patient or family. When a hospice patient transfers to a different program or moves outside a hospice program's service area, the original program should facilitate the patient's transfer by contacting the new program and transmitting the patient's records in a timely manner. Patients covered by the Medicare Hospice Benefit may transfer once during each benefit period.

### Discharge from the Hospice Program

Discharge is an option initiated by the hospice program. It should be exercised only in extraordinary circumstances. Before discharge is considered, the following conditions should exist:

- Every effort has been made and documented to resolve problems and meet the needs of the patient and family.
- Applicable ethical principles have been thoroughly examined, in particular justice, nonmaleficence, nonabandonment, and professional integrity.

Patients may be discharged when:

- The patient and/or family *consistently* indicates their unwillingness to comply with an agreed-upon Plan of Care or compromises the hospice program's standards of care.
- Patient safety issues cannot be resolved.
- Staff safety issues cannot be resolved.
- The patient moves outside the hospice program's service area.

Patients may **not** be discharged just because:

- They cannot pay for services.
- Their illness is expensive to manage.
- They are difficult.
- They require hospitalization for symptom control.

### Revocation of the Medicare Hospice Benefit

Revocation is an option initiated by patients who are covered by the Medicare or Medicaid Hospice Benefit. Patients and families may revoke the benefit at any time during a benefit period. If patients decide to revoke the hospice benefit, traditional Medicare is available immediately. Revocation requirements include the following:

- It must be initiated by the patient and family, not by the program to avoid expensive treatments or difficult situations.
- It must be in writing.
- The hospice program should specify in writing the consequences of revoking the benefit, e.g., the patient or family must make other financial arrangements to continue receiving services the hospice has provided and hospice on-call staff will not be available for emergencies.

### Nonrecertification of Terminal Illness

This option is initiated by the hospice program when a patient covered by the Medicaid Hospice Benefit can no longer be certified as having 6 months or less to live if the disease runs its normal course. A change in the patient's terminal status is the only factor that justifies nonrecertification. When nonrecertification is being considered, the hospice program must:

- Document the recertification process
- Notify the patient and family and primary physician in writing and explain why the patient is no longer considered terminally ill
- Assist the patient with obtaining other, more appropriate services

## Provision of Aggressive Treatments

According to a directive from the Centers for Medicare and Medicaid Services, Medicare-certified hospice programs must provide all covered services that are reasonable and necessary for the palliation and management of the terminal illness. Provided services include palliative radiation and other expensive palliative treatments when symptoms cannot be controlled using other interventions.

*[T]he education and training of physicians and other healthcare professionals fails to provide them with the knowledge, skills, and attitudes required to care well for the dying patient. Many deficiencies in practice stem from fundamental prior failures in professional education. . . . Progress in a clinical field is dependent on its research base. Deficiencies in basic scientific and clinical knowledge affect both the availability of effective palliative therapies and the reimbursement of palliative services. . . . The nation's research establishment should define and implement priorities for strengthening the knowledge base for end-of-life care.*

—Institute of Medicine[44]

*I am convinced that because of the changing emphasis in medicine brought about, in part, because of bioethics, physicians will come to know as much about the person in the coming era as medicine learned about the body in the twentieth century.*

—Eric J. Cassel[13]

## Education

Despite increased societal concern about end-of-life care issues, there is no clear indication that the care of dying patients has improved significantly.[41] Increased lip service is being paid to comprehensive training on end-of-life care, but, in practice, the majority of physicians, medical students, and residents still receive sporadic and unstructured training in the principles and practice of palliative medicine.

In the United States, medical conferences devote very limited space to palliative medicine and research;[102] only five of 126 medical schools surveyed in 1992 offered a separate required course on death and dying,[101] and only 26% of residency programs offer a specific course on end-of-life care.[104] Many physicians, medical students, and residents acknowledge a lack of skill and confidence in the area of palliative medicine and want more education and training on symptom control and managing psychosocial and spiritual concerns.[105,106] In its report on end-of-life care, the Institute of Medicine makes the following points:[44]

- Undergraduate, graduate, and continuing education do not sufficiently prepare health professionals to provide effective care for dying patients.

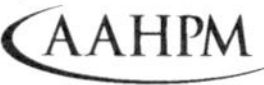

- The education and training of physicians fails to provide them with the attitudes, knowledge, and skills required to care well for dying patients.
- The healthcare community has a special responsibility for educating itself and others about the identification, management, and discussion of the last phase of fatal medical problems.

## World Health Organization's Educational Priorities for Palliative Medicine

The World Health Organization (WHO) focuses on three interrelated domains of palliative medicine education: (1) attitudes, beliefs, and values, (2) knowledge base, and (3) skills.[9] The WHO suggests the following topics as a minimum that should be included in palliative medicine education and recommends requiring demonstrated competence in specific skill areas:[105]

### Attitudes, Beliefs, and Values

- Philosophy and ethics of palliative care
- Personal attitudes about cancer, pain, dying, death, and bereavement
- The complex, interrelated domains of illness: physical, psychological, social, and spiritual
- Interdisciplinary team approach to care
- Family as the unit of care

### Knowledge

- Principles of effective communication
- Pathophysiology of the common symptoms of advanced cancer
- Assessment and management of pain and other symptoms
- Psychological and spiritual needs of seriously ill and dying patients
- Treatment of emotional and spiritual distress
- Psychological needs of the family and other key people
- Availability of community resources to assist patients and their families
- Physiological and psychological responses to bereavement

### Skills

- Setting goals in the physical, psychological, social, and spiritual domains of illness
- Developing a plan of care that addresses the needs of the patient and family
- Monitoring pain and symptom management

## Improving Palliative Medical Education

### Recommendations

To improve education and training on end-of-life care, organizations such as the Institute of Medicine and the American Board of Internal Medicine recommend the following:[44,107]

- Practitioners must hold themselves and their colleagues responsible for using existing knowledge and available interventions to assess, prevent, and relieve physical and emotional distress.
- Educators and other health professionals should initiate changes in undergraduate, graduate, and continuing education to ensure that practitioners have needed attitudes, knowledge, and skills to care for dying patients.
- Medical schools and residency programs should provide comprehensive structured training on end-of-life care.
- Educational materials should be developed that reflect the reality that people die and that dying patients are not people for whom “nothing can be done.”
- Readily available, practical forms for transmitting currently available information about end-of-life care to medical residents, residents, and attending physicians should be developed.
- Palliative care should become a defined area of expertise, education, and research.

### Strategies to Improve Education in Palliative Medicine

To improve education in palliative medicine, Scott and MacDonald suggest several strategies, including the following:[105]

- Concentrate on defining goals and integrating the concepts of palliative medicine throughout the current curriculum, instead of focusing solely on increasing the number of dedicated courses on palliative care
- Help colleagues from other disciplines to incorporate the principles and practice of palliative medicine in teaching, and provide them with case studies and other

teaching materials for use in didactic courses, small-group learning, and other experiences

- Involve faculty role models whose behavior illustrates the principles of palliative medicine
- Illustrate the principles of palliative medicine by including other members of the interdisciplinary team in teaching, e.g., nurses, social workers, and chaplains
- Change student behavior and improve learning by providing hands-on experiences, including guided contacts with patients, families, and hospice staff
- Incorporate well-designed, small-group teaching, seminars, and clinical rotations
- Use educational manuals, videos, computerized instruction, and other informational aids to enhance learning
- Include questions about the principles and practice of palliative medicine in student examinations

### Principles of Undergraduate Medical Education

Billings and Block[108] propose 16 principles for enhancing undergraduate education in palliative medicine, including the following;

- Providing care for dying patients and their families is a core professional task of physicians. Medical schools have a responsibility to prepare students to provide skilled, compassionate end-of-life care.
- At least eight key content areas should be appropriately addressed, including effective communication, pain and symptom management, and accessible and comprehensive home and hospice care.
- Medical education should include the development of positive feelings about dying patients and their families and the physician's role in terminal care.
- Education on death, dying, and bereavement should occur throughout the span of medical education.
- Medical education should foster respect for each patient's personal values and an appreciation of cultural and spiritual diversity.

### Innovative Teaching Methods

Innovative teaching methods increase student awareness of the following:[109]

- Their own preconceived notions about dying and their fears about interacting with dying patients

- The importance of caring relationships in doctor–patient interactions
- The importance of viewing dying patients as real people who live with real families, often in difficult circumstances

### Strategies for Innovative Teaching

Innovative teaching methods incorporate the following strategies:[110]

- Experiential, interactive educational experiences
- Faculty collaboration
- Presentation of lectures and seminars *after* students have interacted personally with patients and listened to their needs and concerns

### Examples of Innovative Teaching Methods

Examples of innovative teaching methods include the following:[44,109]

- Hospice rotations and home visits with members of the interdisciplinary team
- Small-group study of the impact of terminal illness and death on an entire family system, especially with regard to cultural and religious practices
- Role playing communication techniques for sharing bad news and discussing psychosocial and spiritual concerns
- Following patients with advanced illnesses throughout the illness trajectory
- Observing palliative medicine consultations[108]
- Using patient and clinical narratives, literature, and structured opportunities for personal reflection
- Using standardized, simulated patients
- Using role play, videotaped interviews, and discussions of case histories to demonstrate knowledge application in classroom settings[107]

## Research

More than 30 years after Dr. Cicely Saunders proposed research-based care as one of the principles of hospice care, the Institute of Medicine reported the following:[44]

- Current knowledge and understanding are insufficient to guide and support the consistent practice of evidence-based medicine at the end of life.
- The knowledge base for effective end-of-life care has enormous gaps and is neglected in the design and funding of biomedical, clinical, psychosocial, and health services research.
- More and better research is needed to increase understanding of the clinical, cultural, and organizational practices and perspectives that improve care for people at the end of life.
- The nation's research establishment should define and implement priorities for strengthening the knowledge base for end-of-life care, should provide leadership in organizing projects that focus on what is known and not known about end-of-life care, and should propose an agenda for improvements.

## Designing Research Projects

To conserve limited research funds and avoid needless, repeated, burdensome investigations of terminally ill patients and their family members, researchers should:

- Design collaborative projects likely to provide meaningful answers to significant questions[111]
- Give highest priority to problems that cause the greatest suffering[112]
- Carefully consider the following basic questions:[44]

  How significant is the clinical problem? What is its current and future prevalence? What is its burden in terms of morbidity and quality of life? What is its economic burden? How variable are treatments in population subgroups? What symptoms are most distressing? What interventions have been attempted with what results?

  What is the likelihood that the results of the research will affect decisions and outcomes?

  Will the research constructively supplement conclusions from other research?

When designing research projects, key issues such as the following need to be carefully addressed:[112]

- Clarification of the question to be studied
- Choice of treatments and controls
- Selection of the patient sample
- Determination of outcome measures[113]

## Research Challenges in the Terminally Ill Population

Research projects involving terminally ill patients present a number of challenging medical, methodological, economic, and ethical issues, including the following:[111,114]

- Patient vulnerability due to severe, multiple physical and psychosocial symptoms (see UNIPACs Two, Three, and Four)
- Obtaining adequate informed consent due to changes in the patient's mentation and the patient's desire to please hospice caregivers and researchers (see UNIPAC Six)
- Statistical validity of data and recruitment of adequate numbers of patients
- Burdens associated with multiple tests and measurements on already weakened patients
- Drug interactions due to polypharmacy in most terminally ill patients
- Need for careful but innovative use of nonrandomized studies in sometimes uncontrolled settings[44]

Despite significant challenges, well-designed research can build on the results of previous research and lead to better symptom control and increased understanding of the process of dying.

## Areas of Needed Research

Research in palliative medicine is needed to improve patient care. Table 27 lists important examples.

**Table 27: Examples of Needed Research in Palliative Medicine[44,102,112,114,115,116]**

**Pain**

- Treatment of visceral and neuropathic pain
- Identification of receptor-specific opioids
- Improved techniques for drug delivery

**Symptoms Other Than Pain**

- Effective interventions for the cachexia–anorexia–asthenia syndrome
- Effective interventions for cognitive and emotional symptoms

*(Continued)*

**Psychosocial and Spiritual Issues of Patients, Families, and Healthcare Professionals**

- Development of rigorous evaluation strategies and procedures
- Development of clearly articulated outcome measures
- Efficacy of specific therapeutic interventions

**Epidemiology of Dying and Death**

- Clinical pathways of dying, e.g., the duration and patterns of dying, symptom prevalence, functional and cognitive impairment, developmental aspects of illness

**Delivery, Financing, and Improvement of Health Services**

- Effects of national healthcare policies on end-of-life care; integrating palliative care into the continuum of healthcare services
- Effects of organizational structure, financing, and care settings on healthcare costs and health outcomes
- Costs of hospice services and the impact of reimbursement mechanisms on organizational structure, staffing patterns, services, and health outcomes
- Variations in service among hospice programs and their effects on health outcomes. Some hospice programs may provide only one nursing visit per week, while others provide not only multiple weekly visits from nurses, social workers, chaplains, and home health aides, but also continuous infusions of expensive medications and special equipment, such as air flotation mattresses.

**Caregiver Experience and Bereavement**

- Impact of caregiver experiences, demographics, available social supports, and interventions on anxiety, grief, and bereavement outcomes

**Culture, Communication, Perceptions, and Decision Making**

- Effectiveness of specific educational strategies in changing the knowledge, attitudes, and behaviors of healthcare professionals
- Value of case-based learning, role playing, and other innovative educational strategies
- Impact of physician attitudes, skills, and knowledge on health outcomes

*While the specific issues confronting the American hospice movement have changed since those early days, the bedrock challenge remains the same: how to preserve the movement's essential values of compassion and commitment to the real needs of dying patients in the face of growth, financial imperatives and the potential corrupting influence of money.*

—Larry Beresford[117]

*Our love affair with our hospice past has kept us from participating in plans for our future. Instead of idealizing community-based, non-profit care, we should be idealizing the alleviation of pain and suffering. Continued emphasis on the principles and concepts of hospice/palliative care is the only way to ensure that dying patients will receive adequate end-of-life care.*

—Carolyn J. Cassin[56]

*The current patient care delivery system is deficient in regard to the care of the terminally ill. Expertise in pain management often is not available to patients, and comprehensive and enduring care is the exception. We are concerned about providing overly aggressive, unwarranted care, while care that is optimally suited to the dying person's needs is often not available in our health care system or is not covered by insurance.*

—Council on Scientific Affairs, the American Medical Association[118]

Hospice care in the United States is at least a $2 billion industry. Each year more than 400,000 terminally ill patients receive care from more than 2,500 hospice programs, some of which are multimillion dollar corporations employing hundreds of full-time staff.[117] Although hospice care has become a recognized component of the healthcare system, continued provision of comprehensive services for terminally ill patients may be compromised due to factors such as the following:[56]

- The potential impact of millions of aging baby boomers on the entire healthcare system and the need to carefully steward resources to provide appropriate healthcare for all Americans
- The unbundling of hospice services and third-party reimbursement primarily for interventions to relieve physical pain, not for comprehensive, interdisciplinary interventions needed to alleviate the psychological, spiritual, and social components of suffering

- The failure of reimbursement mechanisms to recognize the needs of certain terminally ill patients, e.g., those who are dying of illnesses other than cancer, are less than 65 years of age, or have no primary caregivers
- The reluctance or inability of hospice organizations to address challenges, e.g., barriers to expert palliative care

In the current climate of fiscal restraint, threats to the continued provision of comprehensive services for terminally ill patients have never been greater. However, events such as the following are heightening public interest in compassionate care for the dying:

- The aging of the population and the rise of politically powerful organizations representing the elderly
- Increased concern about the use of physician-assisted suicide to solve patient problems related to the following: depression, anxiety about the future, feelings of powerlessness, fears of becoming a burden to family and friends, and insufficient access to expert palliative care
- Education programs and research sponsored by national groups such as the American Academy of Hospice and Palliative Medicine, the Project on Death in America, the National Institutes of Medicine, the National Hospice and Palliative Care Organization, the American Medical Association, and other professional and lay organizations
- Increased interest in board certification in hospice/palliative medicine, as offered by the American Board of Hospice and Palliative Medicine[119]

# Future Challenges

## Clearly Articulate and Honor the Hospice Message

To ensure the continued provision of comprehensive services for dying patients and their family members, hospice/palliative care organizations must clearly articulate the core values and goals of hospice care and insist that end-of-life care in the United States reflect the hospice message, which encompasses the following:[56]

> When terminally ill patients are supported by an interdisciplinary team of skilled palliative care specialists and volunteers, the last stages of life can become a comfortable and treasured time of new hope and emotional healing. Often, the patient's physical, psychosocial, and spir-

itual suffering can be relieved through effective collaboration among team and family members, who form a caring community in which patients can find new meaning, restored integrity, and a dignified close to life.

## Develop Clinical Outcome Measures

Hospice programs assert that they provide cost-effective interventions that alleviate the suffering of dying patients and family members, but no universally accepted data exist to support this claim. To comply with Saunders's principles of hospice care and to demonstrate the efficacy of palliative interventions, hospice programs must develop robust clinical outcome measures[120] for all domains of care, e.g., physical, emotional, social, and spiritual. Careful research is needed to examine issues such as the following:

- The effectiveness, costs, and benefits of specific interventions in each domain of hospice/palliative care
- Accurate prognosis of terminal illnesses (the NHPCO has published medical guidelines for determining prognosis in selected noncancer diseases, but they have not yet been widely tested)

## Develop and Insist on High Standards of Care

Like the rest of the healthcare system, hospice programs face significant financial challenges. In several states, more than 100 different hospice programs vie for patients in the sometimes lucrative field of hospice care. Traditional nonprofit hospice programs and national for-profit hospice chains now compete not only with one another, but also with national chains of hospitals, nursing homes, and home heathcare agencies offering hospice product lines.[121] In the face of rapid increases in the number of organizations offering hospice-like care and insufficient oversight throughout the healthcare industry, the hospice community should work together to develop the following:[56,117]

- Industry-specific, optimal standards of care and professional competencies
- Clear, objective, valid methods for measuring the quality and effectiveness of hospice services
- Clear methods for evaluating hospice programs to ensure that they are providing comprehensive care and effective interventions that meet the individual needs of individual patients and their families
- Prehospice services for patients needing expert symptom management and emotional and spiritual support, but are not yet ready to forego all curative measures or acknowledge the presence of a terminal illness

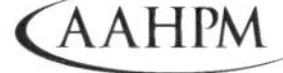

## Reduce Organizational Barriers to Quality Hospice Care

To reduce organizational barriers to care, hospice programs should:

- **Hire staff with adequate clinical skills.** Staff should be able to provide aggressive palliative interventions, e.g., pain control using high-tech pumps, in-depth counseling, and sophisticated spiritual interventions.
- **Hire adequate numbers of staff to provide effective care**. NHPCO has suggested the following caseloads:[18]

  *Registered nurses*: 8 to 12 patients per full-time equivalent (FTE) with an average of 15 to 20 visits per week

  *Social workers*: 20 to 30 patients per FTE with an average of 15 to 25 visits per week

  *Home health aides*: 2 to 15 patients per FTE with an average of 15 to 25 visits per week

  *Chaplains*: 40 to 60 patients per FTE with an average of 15 to 25 visits per week
- **Develop an efficient admission process.** Programs should be able to respond to a request for hospice services within hours, even during evenings and weekends.
- **Encourage careful use of the program's resources so comprehensive care is available for all dying patients**. All members of the interdisciplinary team should serve as patient advocates by providing effective interventions and controlling costs as much as possible.

  *Physicians*: Controlling costs includes (1) prescribing oral medications whenever appropriate, instead of routinely using expensive delivery systems such as transdermal patches, and (2) using less expensive but equally effective treatments whenever possible, e.g., prescribing sorbitol instead of lactulose when an osmotic laxative is required. Simple changes in practice habits may save enough money to provide other vital services, such as spiritual support.

  *Administrators*: Controlling costs could involve reductions in overhead or staff in marketing, public relations, and administration to allow optimum numbers of qualified patient care staff.

## Address Reimbursement Issues

Managed care is a common mechanism for providing healthcare in this country in both public and private sectors.[117] The Medicare Hospice Benefit is an example of managed care, it works within a per diem payment system, financial risks are shifted to the provider, and interventions are guided by a single plan of care.[121] In many cases, the financial returns on investments in managed care programs have been substantial.[122]

Increasingly, corporations are requiring employees and retirees to join managed care programs, which has contributed to rapid increases in enrollment—a nearly tenfold increase since 1976.[123] Little is known about the health outcomes of poor and elderly people enrolled in HMOs. Some researchers voice concerns about issues such as biased patient selection,[124] poor health outcomes,[125] and inadequate patient choice.[126] Medicare and Medicaid are providing incentives for enrolling in a Medicare/Medicaid HMO,[125] which contributed to a doubling of the number of Medicaid beneficiaries enrolled in managed care programs between 1993 and 1994.[127]

To survive, hospice programs must learn to work with managed care in public and private sectors. In general, HMOs are interested in measurable outcomes addressing access, cost, clinical outcomes, and patient satisfaction; they want to purchase cost-effective services that satisfy their customers.[56] Managed care companies are likely to be particularly interested in hospice interventions that support patient or family decisions to forego expensive, futile, inpatient services. To compete, hospice programs must be able to:[56]

- Clearly articulate the unique services that they provide
- Demonstrate the efficacy and cost-effectiveness of their services based on measurable clinical outcomes
- Demonstrate the need for comprehensive palliative interventions, not just medical and nursing interventions[128]

Reimbursement issues that need to be addressed include:

- Restructuring hospice benefits to better serve noncancer patients
- Restructuring the current per diem reimbursement system,[129] which overcompensates for some types of patients, undercompensates for others, and encourages programs to decrease costs and increase profits by providing fewer services for the same per diem
- Pricing hospice services to encourage managed care companies to purchase comprehensive services
- Pricing comprehensive pre-hospice palliative care services
- Educating referral sources so they understand that costs associated with services such as interdisciplinary home visits and the use of continuous infusions in the home setting can save money by decreasing hospitalizations

## Provide Leadership and Work within the Changing Healthcare System

By necessity, hospice care in the United States developed outside the traditional healthcare delivery system, which provided the freedom to develop a comprehensive package of nontraditional but highly effective services to alleviate the suffering of dying patients and their families. However, continued lack of full participation in the healthcare system is hampering the ability of hospice leaders to participate in national discussions about end-of-life care.

In its report on end-of-life care, the Institute of Medicine noted system-wide deficiencies in the healthcare delivery system that interfere with the provision of effective end-of-life care. The Institute recommends that policy makers, consumer groups, purchasers of health care, healthcare providers, and researchers work together to achieve the following goals:[44]

- Develop improved methods for measuring healthcare outcomes and quality of life
- Develop better tools and strategies for improving the quality of care
- Hold healthcare organizations accountable for providing effective end-of-life care
- Develop financing mechanisms that encourage rather than impede comprehensive end-of-life care
- Modify drug prescription laws, regulations, and state medical board policies and practices so that they encourage the appropriate use of opioids to relieve pain

The success of hospice interventions and widespread patient–family satisfaction with hospice services have made end-of-life care look easy. But providing skilled, comprehensive, compassionate care for dying patients is not easy, it is a specialized area of care that demands specific knowledge, skills, and attitudes. To influence national healthcare policy, the hospice community must clearly articulate the following:

- The need to involve hospice/palliative medicine physicians in national decisions about end-of-life care services
- The physical, financial, social, spiritual, and emotional benefits of hospice care for patients, families, and society as a whole
- The costs of poorly managed terminal illnesses on patients, families, and society as a whole, including physical, financial, emotional, social, and spiritual costs
- The need for comprehensive services for dying patients and their family members that encourage care in the home setting
- The need to adequately fund specialized programs that coordinate a full range of services for dying patients and their family members, e.g., hospice programs

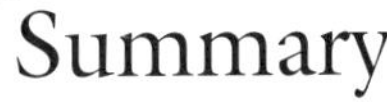

## Summary

For more than three decades, hundreds of thousands of hospice patients and their families have borne witness to the humane and beneficial results of comprehensive hospice/palliative care. In the United States, the more than 25-year experiment with modern hospice care suggests that the process of dying entails more than loss and grief. As long as patients receive comprehensive services, including expert symptom control and emotional and spiritual support, dying can also be a time of increased satisfaction and continued personal growth.[26] Although comprehensive, high-quality hospice care may not be substantially less expensive than conventional care throughout the entire illness trajectory, it offers the most humane way of caring for dying patients. Hospice care can produce significant cost savings during the last months and weeks of life, when conventional care often is most expensive.

Whether or not hospice programs continue to exist in their present form, dying patients and their families continue to need the skilled, comprehensive, interdisciplinary services championed by the hospice movement. We owe the highest level of care to our most vulnerable patients, those who are dying. The means to provide the necessary services are available; all we need is a commitment to caring. Now is the time to honor our commitment, to deliver needed services, and to provide essential education, training, and research.

## The Physician's Role During a Patient's Transition from Curative to Palliative Care

# Henry B. and Doris

Henry is 67-year-old man whose first wife died 3 years ago. Henry has recently retired and married his second wife, Doris. Henry and Doris are just getting settled in their retirement condominium near the golf course when Henry develops a lump on the right side of his neck. He tries to ignore it, but a few weeks later the lump becomes so large that Doris notices it and insists that Henry make an appointment with his physician.

Henry becomes frightened and angry when the physician says the biopsy results indicate lymphoma, but is relieved when the doctor recommends "controlling" the lump with chemotherapy. Because Henry believes that his body needs only a few repairs to get "fixed up" just like his car, he does not complain when the chemotherapy causes nausea, fatigue, and hair loss. Neither Henry, Doris, nor their friends are willing to consider the possibility that Henry might be seriously ill, so they establish a pattern of denial to cope with their fears.

When the tumor on his neck grows larger and a lump appears in his groin, Henry becomes frightened again. He is even more frightened when the physician says the chemotherapy is no longer working. Henry gladly accepts the physician's referral to a regional cancer center, but he is so anxious he does not hear anything else the doctor says during the remainder of the visit.

Doris insists on accompanying Henry to the cancer center. She knows Henry is not telling her everything about his conversation with his physician and realizes that he is very frightened and growing weaker. Henry has not touched his golf clubs for several weeks and eats only small amounts of food. At the cancer center, Henry undergoes numerous tests. Doris wants to attend Henry's meeting with the oncologist so she can hear the test results, ask the doctor's opinion, and plan for the future.

**Question One**

*Assuming that the chances of complete remission are small, which of the following are the oncologist's most appropriate courses of action? Choose all that apply.*

A. Tell Henry not to worry because there are treatments for his condition

B. Share news about the serious nature of the lymphoma and ask Henry and Doris to share their main concerns

C. Tell Henry his condition is terminal and nothing further can be done

D. Suggest various treatment plans, including hospice care.

### Correct Responses and Analysis

The correct responses are B and D. After establishing a trusting relationship, the physician should assess the patient's understanding of the illness, then gently share information that will bring the patient's understanding closer to medical realty. When sharing bad news about a diagnosis, physicians should continually assess the patient's and family's understanding of what is being said and inquire about major concerns. If the patient is terminally ill but not yet psychologically ready to hear bad news about prognosis, hospice care can be still be recommended, with emphasis placed on its home care services, symptom control, and support services for family members, rather than on its services for terminally ill patients. After admission, the hospice team can help Henry and Doris continue the transition from curative to palliative care. (For more information on communicating bad news, see *UNIPAC Five: Caring for the Terminally Ill—Communication and the Physician's Role on the Interdisciplinary Team.*)

Response A is incorrect; it is unlikely that treatments will cure Henry's condition. Offering false reassurance is not only unkind, but is also unethical. Response C is incorrect. Suggesting that nothing can be done is never correct, because symptom control, emotional support, and caring presence are always necessary and appropriate.

**NOTE:** An effective assessment includes open-ended questions about the patient's symptoms and main concerns. For more information on assessing multiple contributors to total pain, see *UNIPAC Two: Alleviating Psychological and Spiritual Pain in the Terminally Ill, UNIPAC Three: Assessment and Treatment of Pain in the Terminally Ill,* and *UNIPAC Four: Management of Selected Nonpain Symptoms in the Terminally Ill.*

## The Case Continues

During a 45-minute appointment, the oncologist performs a careful history and physical and asks Henry about his symptoms. After reviewing the test results with Henry and Doris, the oncologist tells them that the lymphoma is much more serious than expected and then waits for their response. When Henry and Doris remain silent, the physician inquires about their main concerns. Henry says he is most bothered by his lack of appetite and increasing weakness because he wants to get back to the golf course. He is clearly unwilling to think about the implications of his diagnosis.

When asked about her main concerns, Doris looks at Henry, then shakes her head and remains quiet. The oncologist reviews several treatment options, including a new experimental treatment that has many side effects. Henry wants to consider the treatment immediately, but Doris suggests that they investigate further before making a decision. The oncologist concurs with Doris and says that the cancer center can provide more information about the experimental treatment. The oncologist also suggests that Henry and Doris may want to consider hospice care. Henry's face pales. Doris asks for a copy of the hospice brochure she read in the waiting room (while Henry was looking at *Golf Digest*). The oncologist hands Doris a copy of the hospice brochure, schedules a return appointment in 2 weeks, and gives Henry a prescription for megestrol to improve his appetite.

At home, Henry's anxiety about his illness is evidenced by angry comments about the doctor and impatience with his wife. Henry insists, "Of course I'm going to take the new treatment! What other choice do I have!" Doris worries about the experimental treatment because Henry is already very weak. She suggests that unproven treatments can make people feel worse instead of better and may not help the situation. Doris cries when Henry vents his frustrations on her and decides to wait before initiating any further discussion of Henry's illness.

A week later, Henry develops a high fever and increased pain and is too weak to get out of bed. An ambulance takes him to the cancer center emergency room, where IV antibiotics and fluids are started. Then Henry is admitted to the hospital.

**Question Two**

*Which of the following are the oncologist's most appropriate courses of action? Choose all that apply.*

A. Tell Henry he is dying and suggest that he bring his will up to date

B. Meet with Henry and Doris to discuss changes in Henry's condition and inquire about their main concerns

C. Suggest that Henry and Doris meet with someone from a hospice program to discuss home care and symptom control

D. Involve the hospital social worker in discharge planning, including providing information about local hospice programs

### Correct Responses and Analysis

Responses B and D are correct. Meeting with Henry and Doris to discuss their concerns and talk about Henry's changed condition provides another opportunity for the oncologist to help Henry come to terms with his diagnosis and prognosis. Involving the hospital social worker in the meeting provides an opportunity for Henry and Doris to discuss their concerns with someone who may be better able to help Henry consider hospice care as part of his plans for the future.

Responses A and C are incorrect. Telling patients they are going to die before assessing their understanding of the situation, determining how much they want to know, and assessing their readiness to hear bad news is likely to result in their feeling even more abandoned and frightened. This bad news can be delivered more effectively and compassionately. Because Henry has previously expressed dismay at the thought of hospice care, it is more appropriate to wait until his fever and pain are under control to discuss hospice care.

### The Case Continues

Henry's fever resolves after 4 days of antibiotic treatment. The hospital social worker meets with Henry and Doris to discuss discharge planning. When she asks how they are going to manage Henry's care at home, Henry is surprised, because he thought he could stay in the hospital until he was strong enough to care for himself. The social worker mentions hospice care as a possibility and asks if Henry and Doris would be willing to meet with a hospice representative. Doris indicates she would be very interested, but Henry says, "Hospice is for people who are dying and I'm not dying!" Henry says he needs to talk with his oncologist before making any decisions.

The next day Henry is feeling stronger and wants to go home. While talking with Henry and Doris during rounds, the oncologist discovers that the social worker has recommended hospice care and Doris is interested, but Henry is not. Realizing that Henry is still unwilling to consider the implications of his diagnosis, the oncologist confirms that more chemotherapy is not the best choice in this situation. He suggests that Henry at least visit with a hospice representative to discuss how the program can help him remain at home and provide assistance for Doris. Henry hesitantly agrees, then asks if he can see the oncologist again. The oncologist promises to be available by phone to discuss problems that arise, but indicates that Henry's family physician will be resuming Henry's care. The oncologist recommends that Henry and Doris schedule appointments with their family physician and the hospice program. The oncologist also mentions that hospice patients rarely need to return to the cancer center because they receive excellent symptom management. Henry tries to look brave and shakes the physician's hand, saying "Thanks, Doc. Be seeing you."

When they return home, Doris schedules an office visit with their family physician.

**Question Three**

*Which of the following are the most appropriate courses of action for Henry's family physician? Choose all that apply.*

A. Tailor the explanation of hospice services to meet Henry's and Doris's physical and psychological needs

B. Insist that Henry acknowledge his terminal condition

C. Schedule a meeting alone with Doris to discuss Henry's prognosis

D. Acknowledge that Henry and Doris have been through a particularly difficult time and ask about their main concerns

## Correct Responses and Analysis

Responses A and D are correct. Tailoring the explanation of hospice services to the needs of specific patients and families helps them understand how hospice could meet their particular needs. Acknowledging the difficulty of the situation and asking about Doris's and Henry's main concerns may encourage them to share important information.

Response B is incorrect. It is rarely appropriate to insist that patients acknowledge a terminal condition before they are psychologically ready to do so. After receiving training in communication skills, physicians and other healthcare professionals usually become more skilled at helping patients gradually acknowledge the implications of a terminal illness.

Response C can be correct or incorrect depending on the situation. Withholding information from patients at the family's request is not recommended. It excludes patients from participating in healthcare decisions and interferes with completion of the developmental tasks of the dying. Instead, physicians and other team members should normalize the family's concerns about sharing information and model effective communication about death-related concerns. In situations like this one, when patients are unwilling to discuss their condition or consider the implications of their prognosis, providing families with requested information about prognosis acknowledges that, in some cases, families want and need more information or different types of information than patients do. (See UNIPAC Five.)

## The Case Concludes

During the office visit, the family physician meets with Henry and Doris, acknowledges the difficulty of their situation, and mentions that most people in Henry's and Doris's situation feel frightened, uncertain about what to do, and anxious about the best course of action. Then, the physician asks about their main concerns and stops talking long enough for them to consider the question.

Henry breaks the ensuing silence by inquiring about charges for hospice services. The physician reassures Henry that, in his case, hospice services are covered by Medicare and suggests that Henry and Doris make a list of all the questions that they want to ask the hospice representative. The physician notices that Doris's eyes are filled with tears and says, "I see tears in your eyes. Can you tell me something about what is going on with you?" Doris cries quietly for a few minutes, then tells the story of her first husband's death. She says he died while participating in a Phase I trial of a new drug for cancer and both of them suffered terribly during the long, drawn-out process. She says that some of her friends and relatives have used hospice care and have good things to say about it. She asks Henry to consider hospice for her sake.

Henry becomes tearful and agrees to consider hospice, but says he plans to live for a long time. The physician acknowledges that hospice patients may live longer and more independently than expected due to the interventions of an entire team of healthcare professionals. Henry agrees to talk with the hospice representative. The physician calls the hospice office to arrange a referral visit.

Doris follows the physician into the hall and asks about Henry's expected length of life. The physician says it is very difficult to predict how long patients will live and asks Doris about her main concerns. She indicates that Henry's unwillingness to discuss his condition has made it difficult to make needed financial arrangements and rearrange their travel plans. The physician acknowledges Doris's concerns and suggests that she begin financial planning now and that she may need to reconsider any travel plans. Henry's condition could indicate he has weeks left to live, rather than months. Again Doris cries quietly, but thanks the physician for supporting her request for help from a hospice program.

When the hospice representative arrives, she inquires about Henry's and Doris's main concerns, asks for permission to describe some of the services hospice can provide, and tailors the information to meet their needs. She emphasizes the program's focus on keeping patients at home and as independent as possible, on controlling pain and other symptoms so patients can remain as active as possible, and on help for spouses. The representative suggests that Henry try hospice care for a while, then decide if he wants to continue. Henry agrees and says he wants his family physician to act as his attending physician.

Henry is admitted for hospice home care. He receives good symptom management and emotional support from his physician and the entire interdisciplinary team. Gradually, Henry begins to acknowledge his condition and takes charge of the situation by completing a number of tasks, including saying good-by to his family and friends. With aggressive interventions to control his pain and alleviate his psychological and spiritual distress, Henry remains comfortable and alert until he slips into a coma 5 weeks later and dies with Doris by his side. Doris expresses her gratitude to the physician and the hospice program.

## Bereavement Follow-up

Over the next several months, hospice bereavement program volunteers contact Doris at regular intervals and invite her to bereavement support groups. Seven months after Henry's death, a bereavement volunteer notes that Doris is becoming increasingly tearful and unable to sleep. The bereavement coordinator schedules a visit with Doris. During the course of the assessment visit, the coordinator suspects that Doris is experiencing a resurgence of grief over the deaths of Henry and her first husband, a common experience near the first anniversary of a death.

Because Doris is experiencing so much difficulty sleeping, the coordinator suggests that Doris make an appointment with her physician and a bereavement counselor. Doris agrees. Working together, Doris, her family physician, and the bereavement coordinator develop the following plan: Doris will visit with a bereavement counselor to explore her feelings and learn more about the grieving process and will also try to get some regular exercise. The physician will prescribe a short course of medication to make sure that Doris gets some much needed rest. If Doris's situation does not improve within a few weeks, she will make an appointment to see her physician. In any case, she will visit with her physician in 2 months. With this regime, Doris improves. The bereavement coordinator continues to monitor the situation. After 2 months, Doris visits the physician and reports that she is feeling better and is sleeping fairly well without medication. She still misses Henry deeply, but is more involved with life and feels less desperate.

## End-of-Life Care in the Home Setting

# Madeline S.

Madeline S. is a vigorous, independent, 76-year-old retired school teacher who enjoys traveling. She is a widow, and her children, Sally and Mark, are both married and live in distant cities. When Madeline begins to experience fatigue and general discomfort, she visits her physician, who orders chest x-rays that reveal masses on both sides of her lungs. A sputum cytology reveals adenocarcinoma. Madeline's physician informs her of the seriousness of her condition and suggests additional tests to determine which type of chemotherapy is best for her. Madeline says she is not interested in further testing or chemotherapy and thanks the physician for being honest with her. She reports that she has had a good life, does not want heroic treatments, and wants to live the rest of her life as best she can, while remaining in her own home until she dies. Her husband died in great pain in a hospital and she does not want that to happen to her.

The physician prescribes tablets of hydrocodone 5 mg/acetaminophen 500 mg (Vicodin, Lortab) as needed for discomfort, and Madeline does well for about a month. Then she begins to experience considerable nausea and increased, persistent pain. Madeline visits her physician, who notes a large tender liver palpable in the right upper quadrant of Madeline's abdomen. Because she feels so terrible, Madeline reluctantly accepts the physician's recommendation of short-term hospitalization to control her pain and nausea. When the physician asks Madeline if her family should be notified, she blithely replies, "I've already told them everything," but does not reveal further details.

The physician orders metoclopramide (Reglan) 10 mg IV qid, which effectively controls Madeline's nausea, and a patient-controlled analgesia (PCA) pump with 1-mg boluses of morphine to control her pain. Madeline rarely pushes the button. When questioned, she says the morphine is somewhat helpful, but she values her mental clarity and does not want to feel sedated after every dose of morphine. To please her physician, Madeline consents to a CT scan, which reveals multiple large liver metastases and involvement of both sides of her lungs. The source of the adenocarcinoma remains unclear. Madeline continues to refuse chemotherapy and wants to return home. She does not seem to feel hopeless or to be contemplating suicide.

**Question One**

*At this point, which of the following are the most appropriate actions? Choose all that apply.*

A. Insist that Madeline undergo tests to determine the primary site of the adenocarcinoma

B. Discuss hospice care with Madeline

C. Insist that Madeline visit with a psychiatrist to explore her reasons for refusing chemotherapy

D. Switch Madeline to a low-dose, around-the-clock pain medication schedule

### Correct Response and Analysis

The correct responses are B and D. Response B is correct because Madeline is terminally ill and is likely to benefit from hospice services. She needs specialized symptom management and supportive services so that she can remain at home as long as possible. Response D is correct because Madeline can benefit from around-the clock medication to control her pain. When pain persists and is no longer controlled with acetaminophen, aspirin, or another NSAID and a weak opioid, the World Health Organization recommends around-the-clock use of a more potent opioid and needed adjuvant drugs. (See *UNIPAC Three: Assessment and Treatment of Pain in the Terminally Ill.*)

Response A is incorrect. Locating the primary site of Madeline's cancer is unnecessary for effective palliation of symptoms. Subjecting patients who do not want radiation or chemotherapy to additional tests is likely to cause discomfort and increase expenses unnecessarily. Response C is incorrect because Madeline does not appear depressed; patients have every right to refuse unwanted treatments, particularly when they are terminally ill.

## The Case Continues

When the physician mentions hospice and its emphasis on home care, Madeline says she wants to know more about it. When the hospice representative arrives and notes Madeline's IV medicines and the lack of a primary caregiver at home, she indicates that the program cannot admit Madeline, much to the physician's dismay.

The attending physician switches Madeline to oral metoclopramide (Reglan) to control her nausea, and orders transdermal fentanyl (Duragesic) 25 $\mu$g/h to control her pain. Because Madeline is still without a primary caregiver, the physician does not contact the hospice program again and discharges Madeline to a home health care agency.

Within 2 days, the home health care agency nurse calls the physician to report that Madeline's nausea is worse. Madeline can only hold down the metoclopramide (Reglan) tablets occasionally, and she is becoming increasingly confused and less able to care for herself. Madeline decides that the medications are causing her problems, so she stops taking the tablets and peels off the patch. Madeline's mental status improves when the transdermal fentanyl is discontinued, but her pain and nausea worsen considerably. She is taken by ambulance to a hospital emergency room, where she is started on metoclopramide (Reglan) IV 10 mg qid and morphine 0.5 mg every 15 minutes as needed via a PCA pump.

With this regimen, Madeline's nausea improves, but her pain is poorly controlled. Once again, Madeline is alternately uncomfortable or somewhat sedated due to the intermittent doses of morphine. However, she is adamant about returning home and is discharged to the home health care agency on the PCA pump, even though the situation is far from ideal. The apparatus is cumbersome and, once again, Madeline rarely pushes the PCA button during the day because the morphine makes her feels drowsy. She pushes the button during the night, but, because the medication lasts only 1 to 2 hours, she wakes frequently due to pain and is becoming progressively more weary and constipated.

When Madeline's daughter, Sally, calls to talk with her mother, she is alarmed by Madeline's condition. The next day Sally and her brother, Mark, call the home health agency. They are amazed when the nurse tells them that their mother has advanced cancer and is in need of support at home. Madeline had told them only that she was not feeling well and had an appointment with her doctor. When Madeleine discovers that the nurse has divulged confidential information, she is furious. However, she is relieved to see Sally and Mark when they arrive the next day. (See the section, "Confidentiality," in *UNIPAC Five: Caring for the Terminally Ill—Communication and the Physician's Role on the Interdisciplinary Team.*)

Sally and Mark discover that Madeline is able to take small amounts of food and liquid because the metoclopramide (Reglan) IV is controlling her nausea, but she is experiencing considerable discomfort, as well as exhaustion due to lack of sleep. Mark sits up all night and pushes the PCA button every hour so that his mother can sleep, but now he is exhausted. Sally and Mark are even more distressed when they learn that the agency is discontinuing services for Madeline because she has used the allotted number of home care visits that her insurance covers.

On the advice of a friend, Sally and Mark decide to further explore hospice care, and Madeline's physician agrees. They contact a different program. When the hospice admission nurse visits, she tells the family that almost all hospice programs accept patients on IV drugs and work closely with patients who have no primary caregivers so they can receive needed hospice services. She mentions that the Medicare Hospice Benefit does not require a primary caregiver and the NHPCO does not support policies that exclude patients from care. The nurse also mentions that family members sometimes devise rotating schedules to help to provide home care. Madeline is very concerned because her son and daughter are busy professionals and have families of their own, but Sally and Mark assure her that they want to help and will work out something. They also want to honor their mother's wish to remain at home if at all possible. Madeline signs the Medicare Hospice Benefit forms and says she wants her physician to continue serving as her attending physician. Mark returns home. (See the section "Medicare Hospice Benefit" on page 54.)

**Question Two**

*After Madeline is admitted for hospice care, which of the following is the most appropriate action for the hospice medical director?*

A. Ask the hospice home care nurse to call the attending physician and give him a mini-lecture on pain management techniques

B. Do not become involved with Madeline's care because she already has an attending physician

C. Call the attending physician and suggest a consultation visit or recommend medications, delivery routes, and schedules that will improve Madeline's situation

D. Change Madeline's medication without communicating with her attending physician

## Correct Response and Analysis

The correct response is C. Hospice medical directors are responsible for the quality of the medical care of all hospice patients enrolled in the program. Madeline's symptoms are not being adequately controlled. By involving the attending physician, the medical director can establish a collegial working relationship and provide education about symptom management.

Response A is incorrect because medical directors should educate other physicians about symptom control. Although hospice nurses have always played an important role in educating physicians about symptom control and will continue to do so, hospice/palliative medicine physicians have an obligation to share their knowledge. A call from a hospice medical director may receive more attention from a busy physician.

Response B is incorrect because Madeline's symptoms are not being adequately managed and the medical director is responsible for the medical component of the care plans for all hospice patients who are covered by the Medicare Hospice Benefit.

Response D is incorrect; it ignores professional etiquette, and the Medicare Hospice Benefit requires the attending physician's involvement in patient care.

## The Case Continues

The hospice medical director contacts Madeline's attending physician, and recommends custom-made rectal suppositories of dexamethasone 1 mg, hydromorphone 5 mg and metoclopramide (Reglan) 10 mg every 4 to 6 hours, with an additional suppository as needed for breakthrough pain. The medical director also suggests bisacodyl suppositories every other day for constipation. The attending physician agrees and orders the medication, the hospice pharmacist formulates the suppositories, and the hospice home care nurse meets with Madeline and Sally to talk about the benefits of the new medications and the medication schedule.

Madeline, who values her independence, is quite taken aback by the thought of her daughter administering suppositories. The home care nurse acknowledges the common occurrence of initial embarrassment when family members provide personal care, helps Madeline to identify her concerns, and, when the time is right, uses appropriate humor to help Madeline to accept the situation. Sally reassures her mother of her desire to help. (See the section Use Appropriate Humor in *UNIPAC Five: Caring for the Terminally Ill—Communication and the Physician's Role on the Interdisciplinary Team.*)

The nurse also explains that, due to the new dosage of morphine and accumulated sleeplessness, Madeleine is likely to feel drowsy for a few days. She assures Madeline that the feelings of drowsiness are likely to subside and her mental acuity will improve as her body adjusts to the medication. She negotiates with Madeline to try the new regimen for 3 days and gives Madeline an enema to relieve her severe constipation.

Sally convinces Madeline to use 3 to 4 suppositories a day with good symptom relief. At first Madeleine is drowsy, but her mental clarity soon returns and she is more comfortable because her bowels are moving. Sally leaves for home feeling confident that her mother will stay comfortable.

When Mark arrives to relieve Sally, Madeline refuses such personal care from her son and reassures everyone that she can insert the suppositories herself. However, Madeline rarely uses the suppositories and soon experiences a return of nausea and discomfort. Unaware of Madeline's noncompliance, the hospice home care nurse reports Madeline's changed condition to the attending physician. After consultation with the hospice medical director, the attending physician prescribes sublingual soluble morphine tablets to control the apparent breakthrough pain.

The situation continues to deteriorate. Madeline is still not using the suppositories as prescribed so her pain and nausea are increasing and her bowels have not moved in several days. One day, while discussing her feelings about the illness with the social worker, Madeline confesses that she is not using the suppositories as suggested. She is not about to let her son become involved in such personal care. Madeline comments that she much prefers oral medication, but says the bitter taste of the sublingual medication exacerbates her nausea. With Madeline's permission, the social worker reports the situation to the nurse.

During a team meeting later that morning, the hospice nurse suggests injectable medications to control Madeline's nausea, which might increase her ability to tolerate oral pain medication and laxatives. The hospice medical director agrees. The hospice nurse contacts the attending physician, who discontinues the suppositories and orders haloperidol (Haldol) 1 mg SC three times a day for nausea. When Madeline's nausea is controlled, treatment with oral sustained-release morphine tablets and senna tablets twice daily will be initiated to control her pain and constipation.

That afternoon, the hospice nurse inserts a 25-gauge butterfly needle under the skin of Madeline's upper arm and gives the first injection. The nurse shows Mark how to give injections into the injection cap of the butterfly needle and sets up a schedule so Madeline receives three injections a day, with an additional one if she experiences severe nausea. The nurse draws up ten syringes of haloperidol (Haldol) 1 mg and leaves them in the home. Madeline says she much prefers this route to rectal suppositories and experiences considerable relief of her nausea.

Because Madeline's nausea is controlled, she is able to keep down one sustained-release morphine tablet 15 mg twice daily to control her pain, one dexamethasone 2-mg tablet for nausea and appetite, and one senna tablet for constipation. For breakthrough pain, the nurse suggests that Madeline put one of the remaining soluble morphine tablets in a gelatin capsule and swallow it so the bitter taste will not bother her. The nurse also suggests that Mark install hand rails and a raised toilet seat so that Madeline can use the toilet by herself.

Within a few days, this regime is working well. Madeline's appetite improves and her pain is under much better control, with only mild sedation. Mark arranges for a licensed vocational/practical nurse to give the haloperidol injections three times a day. The hospice program arranges for meals on wheels and increases the number of home visits by team members. Hospice volunteers shop for groceries, prepare additional light meals, and provide periodic companionship for Madeline. Mark returns home to check on his family and business.

A week later, the chaplain visits and discovers that Madeleine is quite distressed and worried about burdening her children. She is thinking about committing suicide so her son and daughter will not have to take care of her and jeopardize their jobs. During a called team meeting, which includes a telephone conference with Sally, the team discovers that Sally and Mark are worried because they have used up all their sick-leave time. Sally and Mark want to help and want to respect their mother's wishes, but are not sure what to do. The social worker asks if other family members or friends might be able to help. Mark's wife, Evelyn, agrees to stay with Madeline for a while, even though she and Madeleine have had a somewhat strained relationship. Madeline was very fond of Mark's first wife, who Mark divorced to marry Evelyn.

With help from Evelyn and extra visits from the home care nurse, home health aides, the chaplain, and several hospice volunteers, the situation is resolved for an additional week. Madeline and Evelyn begin to form a better relationship, and Madeline's talk about suicide subsides. Then the on-call nurse receives a call from Evelyn, who reports that Madeline is vomiting and confused. Additional doses of haloperidol (Haldol) have not alleviated her symptoms. When the on-call nurse arrives, Madeline is very nauseated and can no longer hold down the morphine tablets. Madeline also fears she is being poisoned and thinks she is in a sinking boat, where she is desperately trying to find a life jacket.

The attending physician suggests hospitalization, but Madeline refuses. The hospice home care nurse, who has cared for many terminally ill patients, believes that Madeline's symptoms can be controlled in the home setting and suggests an immediate injection of chlorpromazine (Thorazine) 100 mg IM, with a follow-up consultation with the hospice medical director. The attending physician agrees.

**Question Three**

*Which of the following is the most appropriate action for the hospice medical director?*

A. Insist that Madeline be hospitalized for acute symptom management

B. Make a home visit immediately to evaluate the situation and consider providing continuous care services

C. Recommend that Madeline's pain medication be changed to a transdermal patch (Duragesic) 25 $\mu$g/h and continue the haloperidol (Haldol) at 1 mg SC tid

D. Recommend an initial infusion of phenobarbital 130 mg SC hourly, then 600 to 1200 mg per day until Madeline is calm

## Correct Response and Analysis

The correct response is B because a thorough assessment is required. If needed, continuous care is likely to improve Madeline's situation and allow her to remain at home.

Response A is incorrect because Madeline is adamantly opposed to hospitalization and because continuous care in the home and medication adjustments are likely to allow her to remain at home until she dies. Response C is incorrect for the following reasons: the cause of Madeline's distress is very uncertain, the dosage of transdermal fentanyl is lower than the equivalent dose of morphine she was receiving and is unlikely to be effective, and the dosage of haloperidol (Haldol) is also too low. Response D is incorrect in this situation because other, less drastic interventions should be tried first.

## The Case Concludes

The hospice medical director finds that Evelyn is very upset and frightened by Madeline's uncontrolled symptoms. Evelyn says she is exhausted and was forced into an impossible situation and insists that Madeline be transferred to a hospital and then to a nursing home.

Madeline is lying in a soiled bed with her face to the wall. On examination, she grimaces and moans on any movement. Madeline's blood pressure is 110, her respirations are 18, and her temperature is 99°F. She is disoriented to time, but not to person or place. She has moderate jaundice and deep scleral icterus. Her hands have a liver flap on full flexion. Her chest is clear, her heartbeat is rapid and regular, and her abdomen is distended. She has a large tender liver tumor mass palpable 5 cm below the costal margin in the right upper quadrant of her abdomen. She has very few bowel sounds and a large, soft, fecal impaction in her rectum. Her extremities show considerable muscle wasting and decreased skin turgor.

The medical director asks Evelyn for permission to call Mark and Sally and discuss the situation with all three family members. Evelyn burst into tears and agrees. During a three-way conference call, Mark and Sally are very distressed that Madeline's situation has worsened and that she has developed so many problems related to the progression of the cancer: pain, nausea, delirium, anorexia, and restlessness. (See *UNIPAC Four: Management of Selected Nonpain Symptoms in the Terminally Ill.*)

When asked for a recommendation, the medical director suggests continuous care services and more medication for pain and restlessness. The director reminds the family of Madeline's wish to remain home, but says that Evelyn is now exhausted after doing a fine job in a difficult situation. Sally volunteers to pay for sitters to supplement continuous care services and increased home health aide visits provided by the hospice program. Evelyn agrees to stay and maintain the household as long as Madeline's symptoms can be controlled rapidly.

After consultation with the hospice medical director, the attending physician discontinues the sustained-release morphine tablets because Madeline will no longer swallow them and orders an immediate injection of haloperidol 10 mg SC, followed by an SC infusion of Dilaudid 3 mg, Haldol 10 mg, and Versed 5 mg per day. The physician also orders enemas until clear. Along with the continuous care services, this regime controls Madeline's symptoms and her situation improves. However, Madeline now appears to be actively dying and her condition continues to deteriorate.

The hospice nurse and social worker call Sally and Mark and inform them that their mother may be entering the final week or two of life. Madeline is now too weak to get out of bed and sips only liquids. Sally and Mark make arrangements with their employers for special leave under the Family Leave Act.

Madeline now sleeps most of time. When she awakens, she is either somewhat confused or smiling and able to give one-syllable appropriate responses. Madeline sips water only a few times a day. Sally and Mark keep their mother's mouth moistened with ice chips. On two occasions, Madeline experiences increased agitation and tries to climb out of bed, but she is calmed when the hospice on-call nurse gives her an injection of chlorpromazine (Thorazine) 100 mg. The rest of the time Madeline appears to be comfortable. Booster doses of the three-drug SC mixture calm Madeline's periodic restlessness. Five days later, Madeline dies quietly at home with her children at her side.

Although Madeline's course was difficult, her children were proud of themselves for honoring Madeline's wish to remain at home. They were grateful to Evelyn, the attending physician, and the hospice staff for all their support.

## Autonomy and Safety Issues

# David and Elizabeth M.

David is a 78-year-old retired oil business executive who has been married to his wife, Elizabeth, for more than 50 years. David and Elizabeth have no children or close relatives, but they have a very close relationship with one another. Their neighbors are friendly and somewhat helpful but, after so much business-related travel over the years, David and Elizabeth enjoy spending much of their time at home. Their main outside activity is church, which they attend regularly. Elizabeth is somewhat disabled and uses a walker, so David manages the household and stays busy with home improvement projects. He has installed ramps so Elizabeth can walk from the car to the front door without falling.

David smoked cigarettes for 40 years but quit last year for health reasons. He has since been diagnosed with lung cancer. David seems to take the diagnosis in stride, saying, "I guess I can't expect anything else after all those years of smoking. I can't complain; I've had a good life." David's main concern is Elizabeth and what will happen to her after he dies. Elizabeth is quite upset by David's diagnosis; she dreads the thought of living by herself and is not sure how she will manage without his constant help. David agrees to try one round of chemotherapy, but it makes him so weak and nauseated that he discontinues therapy. His only symptom is a constant dull ache in his chest wall, which is managed with one tablet of hydrocodone 5 mg/acetaminophen 500 mg (Lortab) 3 to 4 times a day. To prevent opioid-induced constipation, David also takes a laxative, one senna tablet daily.

David has begun stumbling more often and has fallen several times. One day, Elizabeth finds David lying in the front yard. He dismisses the fall, saying he tripped on a rock, but Elizabeth insists that he see his attending physician. After completing a careful history and physical and discussing the situation with David and Elizabeth, the physician recommends hospice care for David. The services offered by the local hospice program would allow David to remain at home for as long as possible and will provide Elizabeth with much needed help. David and Elizabeth agree.

When the hospice admission nurse arrives, she finds David is alert and oriented, but somewhat forgetful. He gets around the house fairly well, as long as he holds onto furniture. David denies any type of disability. His only complaint is pain on his right side where he was bruised during his last fall. David elects the Medicare Hospice Benefit, and he and Elizabeth sign all the necessary forms.

Because David has few complaints, the team initially focuses on Elizabeth, who is grieving over David's diagnosis and is fearful about the future. Three days after David is admitted for hospice care, Elizabeth calls the hospice on-call nurse and reports that David has fallen and his head is bleeding. When the nurse arrives, she applies pressure to the scalp wound, the bleeding stops, and she is able to get David back in bed. The pain in David's right side is exacerbated by the fall, so the attending physician increases David's pain medication to one tablet of hydrocodone 5 mg/acetaminophen 500 mg (Lortab) 5 times a day, which controls the pain.

During the team meeting the next morning, the hospice physician inquires about the reasons for

David's continuing falls. Nothing seems to explain them, so the hospice physician calls David's attending physician. The attending physician reports that David's gait was somewhat unsteady before his cancer diagnosis and attributes the falls to David's medication. Unconvinced, the hospice physician suggests that the hospice nurse check David's mental status, gait, and blood pressure both lying and standing. The attending physician agrees. The assessment reveals that David is alert and friendly, but his memory is somewhat impaired, he has a broad-based shuffling gait, and his blood pressure falls only 5 points from lying to standing, from 135 to130, none of which explain the falls. The hospice volunteer coordinator arranges for a volunteer to install additional handrails in the bathroom and tack down loose carpet.

A week later, Elizabeth hears a loud crash and discovers that David has fallen again. He is lying on the floor, moaning. Elizabeth is very upset and immediately calls the hospice program.

**Question One**

*At this point, which of the following is the most appropriate response for David's attending physician?*

A. Insist that David revoke the Medicare Hospice Benefit because the hospice program is not coping with David's increasing disability

B. Reevaluate David's condition

C. Prescribe a heavy sedative so that David will not be able to get out of bed

D. Tell Elizabeth not to worry about David because he is going to die soon anyway

## Correct Response and Analysis

The correct response is B. An evaluation of David's condition and his gait-related problems may suggest interventions that will improve the situation. The other responses are incorrect. Revoking the benefit will result in loss of much needed hospice services and emotional support. Prescribing a heavy sedative is premature; David still experiences good quality of life much of the time. Telling Elizabeth not to worry about a very distressing situation is unhelpful and counterproductive.

## The Case Continues

The hospice physician calls David's attending physician and offers to make a home visit, but the attending physician wants to admit David to the hospital. David is transferred to a hospital that contracts with the hospice program. During the hospital admission process, an intern and resident notice David's multiple bruises, the laceration on his skull, and his unsteady gait and order four-point restraints. When the hospice nurse arrives, she finds David very upset and agitated, with his wrists and ankles lashed to the bed rails.

**Question Two**

*At this point, which of the following is the best response for the hospice nurse?*

A. Request heavy sedation for David to calm his agitation

B. Suggest that David accept the situation

C. Remove David from the hospital and cancel the hospice contract with the hospital

D. Involve the hospice medical director and the attending physician

## Correct Response and Analysis

The correct response is D. Because the hospice program is responsible for managing the patient's care, both the medical director and attending physician should be involved. Together they may be able to resolve the conflict with the hospital. Responses A and B are incorrect because David has every right to be upset and agitated about the restraints. Response C is incorrect because David's condition does need to be thoroughly evaluated and canceling the contract will not resolve the situation.

## The Case Continues

The hospice nurse immediately meets with the unit director and explains that David has been getting along fairly well at home and has been admitted for evaluation, not restraints. The unit director explains that liability issues necessitate restraints.

Recognizing that the calamitous situation is unlikely to be resolved without help from the hospice medical director and David's attending physician, the hospice nurse places urgent calls to both. The attending physician arrives and performs a careful history and physical, during which David is asked to move his finger from the attending's finger to his own nose and back again. It is apparent that David has lost the ability to accomplish this task. Nor can he turn his hand over rapidly from side to side, both signs that David's cerebellum functioning is compromised, most likely due to metastases to the brain. The attending physician suggests a CT scan of David's brain, but David and Elizabeth refuse because the results of the test would not change the therapy.

After consulting with the hospice medical director, the attending physician orders a physical therapy consult to evaluate David's gait, prescribes dexamethasone 4 mg twice a day, and negotiates a compromise with the unit director.The restraints will be removed, the bed rails will stay raised, and David will sit in a Neuro-chair during the day, if he agrees not to climb out of bed.

When the hospice social worker visits the next day, she finds David very depressed. He is distressed because he has to wear diapers that are not changed often enough, and he is worried about Elizabeth. The social worker encourages David to remain in the hospital one more day to take advantage of the physical therapy consult and promises to check on Elisabeth and arrange more help if needed. That night, David has difficulty sleeping due to the steroids and becomes more confused in the unfamiliar hospital environment. He tries to get to the bathroom, falls out of bed, and is found on the floor of the hospital. The x-rays reveal no fractures, but David is sore and bruised. It is apparent that the dexamethasone is not going to immediately improve David's ability to ambulate.

During the physical therapy evaluation, the therapist finds that David can transfer independently from his bed to a walker and can use the walker appropriately most of the time. However, on two occasions, David moved too close to the front of the walker and would have fallen if the physical therapist had not been there to catch him. David is no longer sure which year it is, but insists on going home.

**Question Three**

*At this point, which of the following is the attending physician's best response?*

A. Transfer David back to home, with intensive follow-up and increased hospice services

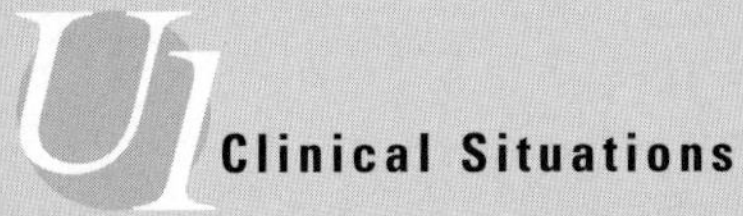



B. Encourage David to remain in the hospital for physical therapy treatments

C. Discontinue all pain medications to improve David's mental acuity

D. Discontinue hospice services because David's condition makes his home environment unsafe

### Correct Response and Analysis

The correct response is A. Every attempt should be made to honor David's wishes. Increased hospice services may allow David to remain at home until he dies. The other responses are incorrect. B is incorrect because encouraging David to remain in the hospital is unlikely to be productive. In addition, a significant number of patients with conditions similar to David's develop delirium while in the hospital, from which they are unlikely to recover. C is incorrect because David's pain medication is unlikely to be causing his confusion and discontinuing it will result in increased pain. D is incorrect because increased hospice services may allow David to remain at home safely until he dies.

### The Case Continues

David is transferred back home. Because David's fall in the hospital increased his pain, his medication is increased to oxycodone 5 mg with acetaminophen 325 mg (Percocet) one tablet q 4 hours. The dexamethasone is discontinued because it is neither alleviating David's increasing weakness nor his unsteadiness, both of which are being caused by progressive disease. The dexamethasone also stimulated David's appetite, which was exacerbating safety problems because he was getting up several times during the night to eat. This increased his risk of falling and interfered with Elizabeth's ability to sleep through the night.

To avoid burdening Elizabeth, David tries desperately to care for himself. He toilets himself and fixes his own food, even at the risk of falling. Elizabeth is torn by conflicting emotions; she is very worried about David's safety and wonders if he would be better off in a nursing facility, but she wants to be with him during the final stage of his life and wants to honor his wish to remain at home. She also hopes he will die without suffering for too long, but knows she will miss him terribly and is concerned about what will happen to her after he dies.

At the team meeting, nursing home placement for David is suggested due to safety concerns and the burdens on Elizabeth. The chaplain, who has visited with David several times, reports that David's worst fear is being placed in a nursing home away from Elizabeth. David has said he would kill himself rather than go to a nursing facility. The chaplain suggests that any intervention the team can devise to keep the couple together would be the most life-enhancing service that the program could offer. The hospice nurse suggests in-home physical therapy to improve David's ability to use his walker, a bedside commode for use at night, and installation of a toilet seat with rails. The social worker suggests meals on wheels. The home health aide recommends daily visits to help Elizabeth keep David clean. The volunteer coordinator suggests increased volunteer help, both from the hospice program and from David's church, to help with grocery shopping and installing a raised toilet seat. The attending physician agrees with the proposed interventions.

With increased care, David's situation improves and he and Elizabeth enjoy their time together for the next 2 weeks. Then David falls again while wandering around the house at night. On questioning, David says that he has always gotten up several times during the night, so his behavior is not unusual. He does not complain about lack of sleep. The hospice nurse suggests a hypnotic at bed time to keep David asleep through the night, but the attending physician fears that the medication will make David more unsteady if he awakens and tries to walk.

During the next 2 weeks, David's situation deteriorates. When inpatient care is suggested, David begs Elizabeth not to send him away. David is now so weak he can barely get from bed to the bedside commode. He suddenly develops more pain in his chest and head and starts seeing people who are not there. The hospice nurse describes David's situation to the attending physician, who orders sustained-release morphine 30 mg twice a day, with oxycodone 5 mg with acetaminophen 325 mg (Percocet) as needed for breakthrough pain, and senna two tablets twice a day. The physician also orders haloperidol (Haldol) 2 mg in AM and 2 mg at night. When the hospice nurse suggests that more sedation at night might be helpful, the physician agrees and increases the haloperidol (Haldol) to 4 mg at night.

These interventions are very helpful. David is no longer in pain and he sleeps comfortably through the night. With frequent visits from the hospice volunteers and home health aides, Elizabeth is able to care for David at home. Three days later, David's situation again takes a rapid turn for the worse. He is very restless and uncomfortable.

**Question Four**

*At this point, which of the following is the best intervention?*

A. Prescribe an infusion of phenobarbital to induce unconsciousness

B. Initiate continuous care and switch from haloperidol (Haldol) to thioridazine (Mellaril) 25 mg in the morning and 75 mg at bedtime

C. Suggest physician-assisted suicide

D. Discontinue the morphine because it may be contributing to the pain in David's head

## Correct Response and Analysis

The correct response is B. The extra nursing care provided by continuous care in the home setting will help to ensure that David's symptoms are closely monitored and carefully controlled and will provide much needed support for Elizabeth. Switching from haloperidol (Haldol) to thioridazine (Mellaril) may alleviate David's restlessness and make him more comfortable.

Response A is incorrect because it is premature. Using an infusion of phenobarbital to induce unconsciousness may be appropriate when severe symptoms cannot be managed in any other way but, in this case, thioridazine (Mellaril) should be tried first because it may control David's restlessness and leave him conscious enough to continue interacting with Elizabeth. Response C is incorrect because physician-assisted suicide is outside the scope of this program's interventions. Response D is incorrect because discontinuing the morphine is unlikely to improve his mental clarity and may worsen his head pain.

## The Case Concludes

The thioridazine (Mellaril) effectively controls David's restlessness. He sleeps almost 18 hours a day, but can be aroused for meals and for brief visits with his wife, neighbors, church friends, and the hospice staff. He gives one-word responses, then drifts back to sleep. In David's case, the normal somnolence that usually occurs during the dying process is exacerbated by the Mellaril, but the increased sedation is helpful because it controls David's restlessness. It also reduces his desire to get out of bed, which is helpful because his weakened condition almost guarantees that he will fall. David occasionally eats a few bites of soft food, is bathed daily by hospice home health aides, and is closely monitored by continuous care nurses until his condition stabilizes.

Elizabeth is grieving, but is coping reasonably. A week later, David looses the ability to swallow. With assistance from the home health aides, Elizabeth gives David sustained-release morphine rectally, in addition to suppositories of chlorpromazine (Thorazine) 50 mg in AM and 100 mg at night and a bisacodyl suppository tablet every other day for constipation. Two days later, David dies comfortably with Elizabeth and a hospice volunteer by his side.

The hospice social worker and Elizabeth's church friends arrange for her to move to an assisted living facility where she knows some of the residents. The hospice program provides bereavement services for the next year. On multiple occasions Elizabeth tells the bereavement counselor how important it was for her to be with David during the final weeks of his life and to honor his wish to remain at home until he died. Elizabeth is very grateful to the hospice program and the attending physician for honoring David's wishes.

# Pretest Correct Answers

1. C
2. C
3. C
4. A
5. C
6. B
7. C
8. A
9. D
10. C
11. B
12. B
13. C
14. B
15. A
16. D
17. B
18. D
19. C
20. D
21. A
22. C
23. D
24. B

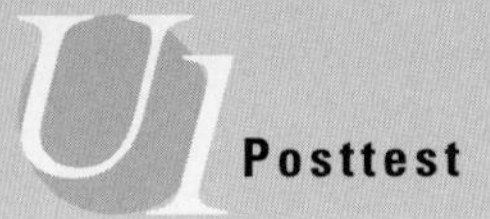

## Posttest

Read each item and circle the one correct response to each item on the detachable answer sheet at the back of the book.

1. **The principles of hospice care developed by Dr. Cicely Saunders include all the following except which one?**

   A. Research is inappropriate in hospice settings.

   B. A team of clinical professionals is needed to control symptoms.

   C. Home care is a vital component of hospice care.

   D. Teaching all aspects of terminal care is an essential component of a hospice physician's responsibilities.

2. **The rules for making prudent judgments include all the following except which one?**

   A. Physicians should refrain from offering an opinion about a treatment because they may influence a patient's choice.

   B. Physicians should pay increased attention to patient vulnerability.

   C. Physicians should maintain a healthy respect for moral ambiguity.

   D. Physicians should encourage patient autonomy.

3. **In the United States, all the following are barriers to palliative care for terminally ill patients in the home setting except which one?**

   A. Lack of adequate insurance coverage

   B. Inadequate numbers of hospice programs in most cities

   C. Lack of physician skill in pain management and communication

   D. Lack of coordination of services for nonhospice patients

4. **All the following statements about the Medicare Hospice Benefit are true except which one?**

   A. To receive the Medicaid Hospice Benefit for coverage of a terminal illness, patients waive traditional Medicare hospital coverage for the terminal illness.

   B. The Medicare Hospice Benefit pays hospice programs at a per diem rate to cover all healthcare costs related to the terminal diagnosis, including prescription medications.

   C. After choosing the Medicare Hospice Benefit, patients are still covered by traditional Medicare Part A for problems unrelated to the terminal diagnosis.

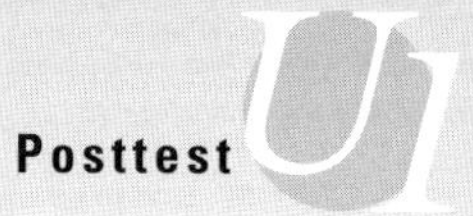

D. More than 80% of elderly patients have chosen the comprehensive coverage offered by the Medicare Hospice Benefit.

**5. All the following statements about the Medicare Hospice Benefit are true except which one?**

A. The benefit pays a per diem that covers all medicines, biologicals, durable medical equipment, and medical supplies needed to palliate symptoms related to the terminal illness.

B. The benefit includes coverage for services from home health aide and homemakers.

C. The benefit covers the cost of a patient's room and board in a nursing home.

D. The benefit covers respite stays for patients to relieve family member distress.

**6. All the following statements about Medicare Hospice Benefit reimbursement for physicians are true except which one?**

A. An attending physician bills Medicare Part B for professional services related to chemotherapy or radiation therapy.

B. A consultant physician bills the hospice program directly for professional services related to chemotherapy or radiation therapy.

C. The attending physician bills Medicare Part A for the cost of chemotherapy drugs.

D. When consulting physicians bill the hospice program for professional services, the program is reimbursed by Medicare Part A for 100% of the Medicare allowable amount.

**7. All the following statements about hospice program polices are true except which one?**

A. It is permissible to deny hospice services to terminally ill patients who threaten the personal safety of hospice staff.

B. Hospice programs can ethically discharge patients whose symptoms are too expensive to manage.

C. Medicare-certified hospice programs must provide all covered services included in the patient's Plan of Care that are reasonable and necessary for the palliation and management of a terminal illness.

D. To improve access for underserved populations, hospice program policies should train staff to communicate effectively with patients from various ethnic groups and religious traditions.

8. **All the following are essential components of hospice/palliative medicine except which one?**

   A. Alleviating the suffering of patients and family members

   B. Helping patients and families make the transition from illness to death to bereavement

   C. Focusing solely on the physical aspects of suffering

   D. Participating in the patient's search for meaning and hope

9. **All the following statements about the responsibilities of physicians practicing hospice/palliative medicine are true except which one?**

   A. Provide guidance and support as patients make the transition from curative to palliative care.

   B. Provide information about diagnosis, prognosis, and treatment options.

   C. Give selflessly to patients and their family members, staff, and team members.

   D. Participate in team meetings.

10. **All the following are barriers to effective end-of-life care except which one?**

    A. Misconceptions about opioids on the part of many healthcare professionals, e.g., opioids cause addiction

    B. Lack of effective medications to control pain

    C. Lack of medical school emphasis on end-of-life care

    D. The widespread belief among physicians that there is nothing they can do when patients are terminally ill

11. **All the following statements about the costs of hospice care are true except which one?**

    A. Definitive studies have proved that hospice care reduces healthcare costs throughout the illness trajectory.

    B. Hospice care and the use of advance directives may save 25% to 40% of healthcare costs during the last month of a patient's life.

    C. Because comprehensive hospice/palliative care involves complex, interdisciplinary interventions, it may not be less expensive than conventional care throughout the illness trajectory.

    D. Aggressive palliative interventions may require large quantities of expensive medications, radiation therapy, or surgical interventions.

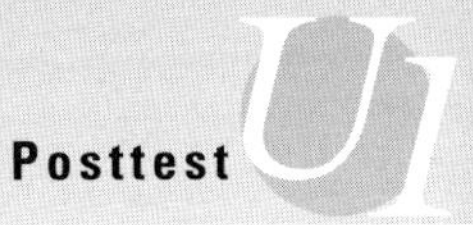

**12. All the following statements about the Medicare Hospice Benefit are true except which one?**

A. The revised benefit consists of two 90-day periods followed by an unlimited number of 60-day periods.

B. Patients may revoke the hospice benefit at any time, but revocation results in the loss of all remaining days in that benefit period.

C. When patients revoke the hospice benefit, traditional Medicare Part A is immediately available to them.

D. At the end of each benefit period, patients are automatically eligible for continuation of the hospice benefit.

**13. All the following statements about Medicare Hospice Benefit reimbursement for physician services are true except which one?**

A. Administrative services provided by physicians employed by the hospice are not included in the hospice program's per diem rate and can be billed separately.

B. Physicians who are hospice employees or who provide direct patient care services under arrangement with the hospice bill the hospice program directly for professional services and are reimbursed at an agreed-upon rate.

C. Attending physicians who are not hospice employees but provide direct patient care services bill Medicare Part B for professional services just as they would for nonhospice patients.

D. Consulting physicians who provide patient care services bill the hospice program directly for professional services and are reimbursed by the program at an agreed-upon rate.

**14. All the following statements about ethical issues related to hospice/palliative care are true except which one?**

A. Increasing religious and cultural diversity requires careful attention to the values, needs, and concerns of each patient.

B. When news of a life-threatening illness affects a patient's ability to make decisions, the physician should help the patient to articulate his or her beliefs, values, and goals.

C. Physicians are obligated to honestly and compassionately tell patients as much as they want to know about their diagnosis and prognosis.

D. Patients are obliged to participate in research projects that may improve hospice/palliative care for others.

**15. All the following definitions are true except which one?**

A. Palliative care is the term used to describe whole-person care provided by an interdisciplinary team of healthcare professionals.

B. Palliative treatments enhance comfort and improve a patient's quality of life.

C. Therapies such as bone marrow transplantation or craniotomy for resection of metastases cannot be palliative interventions.

D. Hospice programs provide palliative care to terminally ill patients 24 hours a day, 7 days a week in both home and facility-based settings.

**16. The NHPCO Standards of Care for Hospice Programs include all the following except which one?**

A. The hospice interdisciplinary team collaborates continuously with the patient's attending physician.

B. Hospice programs can offer fewer services to patients residing in nursing facilities.

C. Hospice programs offer palliative care services to terminally ill patients regardless of their diagnosis, availability of a primary caregiver, or ability to pay.

D. Hospice care services are available 24 hours a day, 7 days a week.

**17. All the following statements about Dr. Elizabeth Kübler-Ross are true except which one?**

A. Her book, *On Death and Dying*, was a best-seller and sparked widespread interest in the care of dying patients.

B. She described the conspiracy of silence that surrounds dying people.

C. She believed that patients always experience five stages of dying in exactly the same order: denial, anger, bargaining, depression, and acceptance.

D. She interviewed dying patients about their reactions to dying.

**18. All the following statements about ethical issues in the home setting are true except which one?**

A. Patients have a right to know their diagnosis, prognosis, and treatment options.

B. Physicians can share confidential patient information with other members of the interdisciplinary team without the patient's consent.

C. Treating the patient's symptoms just to relieve family distress can be an ethically correct choice in some situations.

D. Patients should not be sedated against their will.

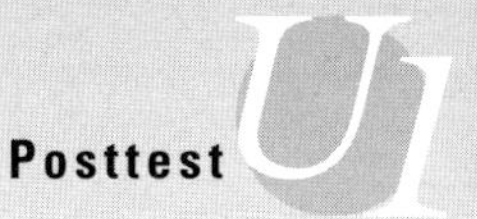

**19. All the following statements about patient eligibility for the Medicare Hospice Benefit are true except which one?**

A. In most cases, the patient must be 65 years of age or older and be eligible for Medicare Part A.

B. The patient must have a primary caregiver in the home.

C. In most cases, the patient must be certified as terminally ill by two physicians.

D. Care related to the patient's terminal illness must be provided by a Medicare-certified hospice program.

**20. All the following statements about the Medicare Hospice Benefit are true except which one?**

A. The benefit provides per diem reimbursement based on four levels of care: routine home care, continuous home care, general inpatient care, and respite care.

B. Continuous home care is for crisis management of acute symptoms so patients can remain at home; at least 51% of the care must require the services of licensed nurses.

C. The per diem rate for routine home care is paid regardless of the number of services provided on a particular day.

D. Medicare sets no limits on reimbursement for needed services.

**21. All the following statements about the palliative model of care are true except which one?**

A. A palliative intervention is indicated if it controls symptoms and relieves suffering.

B. Emphasis is placed on knowing the patient's values, beliefs, and concerns.

C. The primary goal is cure of the patient's disease.

D. The subjective experiences of patients are valued as highly as objective data from laboratory tests.

**22. All the following statements about hospice/palliative care are true except which one?**

A. Each patient's beliefs, values, and concerns should be respected regardless of race, religion, sexual orientation, or financial status.

B. Hospice/palliative care interventions should be based on the results of careful research.

C. People, especially those who are suffering, rarely need help articulating their needs, values, concerns and fears.

D. Skillful interdisciplinary interventions can help to alleviate suffering.

**23. All the following statements about Dr. Cicely Saunders are true except which one?**

A. Dr. Saunders is usually credited with developing the art and science of modern hospice care.

B. Dr. Saunders founded the world-renowned St. Christopher's Hospice in England.

C. Dr. Saunders developed the concept of total pain, which describes the all-encompassing physical, emotional, spiritual, and social pain experienced by many dying patients.

D. Dr. Saunders was more concerned with general concepts than with the details of patient care or research.

**24. All the following statements about managing symptoms of advanced cancer in patients in the home setting are true except which one?**

A. When insomnia is a problem for a confused patient, major tranquilizers such as thioridazine (Mellaril) or chlorpromazine (Thorazine) may be more useful than benzodiazepine hypnotics.

B. When convulsions or acute delusional states are a problem, most families can learn to use subcutaneous routes to deliver medications such as phenobarbital or haloperidol.

C. When fecal incontinence is a problem, use osmotic laxatives like lactulose and sorbitol.

D. When bleeding is a problem, avoid NSAIDs and Coumadin, and control hypertension aggressively.

# References

[1]Stoddard S. *The Hospice Movement: A Better Way of Caring for the Dying.* New York: Stein and Day Publishers; 1978. (Revised version available: Stoddard S. *The Hospice Movement: A Better Way of Caring for the Dying.* New York: Vintage Books; 1992.)

[2]Meade M. *Throw yourself like seed.* Pacific Grove, California: Oral Tradition Archives;1996.

[3]von Gunten CF, Muir JC. Palliative medicine: an emerging field of specialization. *Cancer Invest.* 2000;18((8):761–767.

[4]Callahan D, Parens E. The ends of medicine: shaping new goals. *Bull NY Acad Med.* 1995;72:95–117. Cited by: Fox E. Predominance of the curative model of medical care: a residual problem. *JAMA.* 1997;278(9):761–763.

[5]Pellegrino ED, Thomasma DC. *Helping and Healing.* Washington, DC: Georgetown University Press;1997:27. Cited by: Fox E. Predominance of the curative model of medical care: a residual problem. *JAMA.* 1997;278(9):761–763.

[6]Fox E. Predominance of the curative model of medical care: a residual problem. *JAMA.* 1997;278(9):761–763.

[7]Cassell EJ. *The Nature of Suffering and the Goals of Medicine.* New York: Oxford University Press; 1991:33–34.

[8]Byock IR. The nature of suffering and the nature of opportunity at the end of life. *Clin Geriatric Med.* 1996;12(2): 237–252.

[9]*Cancer Pain Relief and Palliative Care: Technical Report Series 804.* Geneva: World Health Organization; 1990.

[10]Doyle D, Hanks G, MacDonald N. Introduction. In: Doyle D, Hanks G WC, MacDonald N, eds. *Oxford Textbook of Palliative Medicine.* New York: Oxford University Press; 1993:3–8.

[11]American Board of Hospice/Palliative Medicine. *Certification Examination in Hospice and Palliative Medicine.* New York: Professional Testing Corporation. Brochure.

[12]*Standards of a Hospice Program of Care.* Arlington, Va: National Hospice Organization; 1993.

[13]Cassel EJ. The importance of understanding suffering for clinical ethics. *J Clin Ethics.* 1991;2(2):81–82.

[14]Rusnack B, Schaefer S, Moxley D. Safe passage: social work roles and functions in hospice care. *Social Work in Health Care.* 1988;13:3–19. Cited in: Rusnack B, Schaefer SM, Moxley D. Hospice: social work's response to a new form of social caring. *Social Work in Health Care.* 1990;15(2):95–118.

[15]Saunders C, ed. *The Management of Terminal Disease.* London: Edward Arnold Ltd; 1978:195–202.

[16]Cohen SR, Mount BM, Strobel MG, Bui F. The McGill Quality of Life Questionnaire; a measure of quality of life appropriate for people with advanced disease. A preliminary study of validity and acceptability. *Palliat Med.* 1995;9(3):207–219.

[17]Tulsky JA, Steinhauser KE, Bosworth HB, Clipp EC, McNeilly M, Christakis NA. Assessment of a new instrument to measure quality of life at the end of life. *J Palliat Med.* 2002;5(1):206. Abstract.

[18]National Hospice Organization. Hospice services guidelines and definitions. *Hospice J.* 1996;11(2):65–73.

[19]Jonsen AR, Siegler M, Winslade WJ. *Clinical Ethics.* New York: Macmillan Publishing Co; 1982.

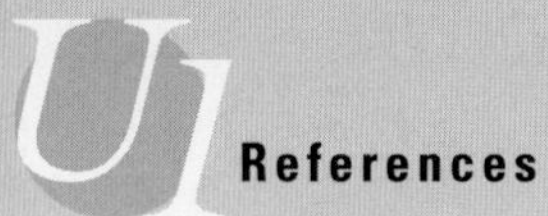



[20]von Gunten CF, Martinez J. Role of palliative medicine in cancer patient care. *Cancer Treat Res.* 2000;102:65–76.

[21]Saunders C, Baines M. *Living with Dying.* New York: Oxford University Press; 1989.

[22]Delbanco TL. Enriching the doctor–patient relationship by inviting the patient's perspective. *Ann Intern Med.* 1992;116(5): 414–418.

[23]Bailey JE. Asklepios: ancient hero of medical caring. *Ann Intern Med.* 1996;124(2):259–263.

[24]MacDonald N. The interface between oncology and palliative medicine. In: Doyle D, Hanks G W C, MacDonald N, eds. *Oxford Textbook of Palliative Medicine.* New York: Oxford University Press; 1993:11–17.

[25]Hallenbeck JL. Cultural considerations of death and dying in America. Presented at the 8th Annual Assembly of the Academy of Hospice Physicians; June 12–16, 1996; Snowbird, Utah.

[26]Byock I. *Dying Well: The Prospect for Growth at the End of Life.* New York: Riverhead Books; 1997.

[27]Thomasa DC. Beyond medical paternalism and patient autonomy: a model of physician conscience for the physician–patient relationship. *Ann Intern Med.* 1983,98:243–248.

[28]Bennahum DA. The historical development of hospice and palliative care. In: Sheehan DC, Forman WB. *Hospice and Palliative Care.* Sudbury, Mass: Jones and Bartlett; 1996.

[29]Morris, D.B. Collaborations: writers and the health-care professional. Presented at the 9th Annual Assembly of the American Academy of Hospice and Palliative Medicine. Chicago, Illinois. June 25–28, 1997.

[30]Seplowin VM, Seravalli E. The hospice; its changes through time. In: Kutscher AH, Klagsbrun SC, Torpie RJ, DeBellis R, Hale MS, Tallmer M, eds. *Hospice USA.* New York: Columbia University Press; 1983.

[31]Craven J, Wald F. Hospice care for dying patients. *Am J Nurs.* 1975;75:1816–1822. Cited by: Campbell L. History of the hospice movement. *Cancer Nurs.* 1986;9(6):333–338.

[32]Campbell L. History of the hospice movement. *Cancer Nurs.* 1986;9(6):333–338.

[33]Walsh TD, Saunders CM. Hospice care; the treatment of pain in advanced cancer. *Cancer Research.* 1984;89:201–211.

[34]Kerr D. Mother Mary Aikenhead, the Irish Sisters of Charity and Our Lady's Hospice for the Dying. *Am J Hospice Palliat Care.* 1993;9(3):13–20.

[35]Storey P. Goals of hospice care. *Texas Medicine.* 1990:86(2):50–54.

[36]Kübler-Ross E. *On Death and Dying.* New York: MacMillan; 1969.

[37]National Hospice Organization. *Hospice Fact Sheet.* Arlington, Va: National Hospice Organization; December 10, 2001.

[38]Cassel CK, Vladeck BC. ICD-9 code for palliative or terminal care. *N Engl J Med.* 1996;335(16):1232–1233.

[39]Callahan D. *The Troubled Dream of Life; In Search of a Peaceful Death.* Portland, Ore: Touchstone Press; 1996.

[40]Horgan J. Seeking a better way to die. *Scientific American.* May, 1997:100–105.

[41]Cassel CK. Overview on attitudes of physicians toward caring for the dying patient. In: *Caring for the Dying: Identification and Promotion of Physician Competency.* Philadelphia, Pa: American Board of Internal Medicine; 1996:1–4.

[42]Schechter, GP. Professionalism in providing end-of-life patient care. In: *Caring for the Dying: Identification and Promotion of Physician Competency.* Philadelphia, Pa: American Board of Internal Medicine; 1996:5–7.

[43]Twycross RG. Why palliative medicine? *Henry Ford Hosp Med J.* 1991;39(2):77–80.

[44]Field MJ, Cassel CK, eds. *Approaching Death: Improving Care at the End of Life.* Report by the Committee on Care at the End of Life. Institute of Medicine. Washington, D.C.: National Academy Press; 1997.

[45]Foley KM. Palliative medicine, pain control, and symptom assessment. In: *Caring for the Dying: Identification and Promotion of Physician Competency.* Philadelphia, Pa: American Board of Internal Medicine. 1996:11–26.

[46]Jacox A, Carr DB, Payne R, et al. *Management of Cancer Pain. Clinical Practice Guidelines No. 9. AHCPR Publication No 9-0592.* Rockville, Md. Agency for Health Care Policy and Research, U.S. Department of Health and Human Services, Public Health Service, March, 1994.

[47]SUPPORT. The SUPPORT clinical investigators. A controlled trial to improve care for seriously ill hospitalized patients. *JAMA.* 1995;274:1591–1598.

[48]Council on Scientific Affairs, American Medical Association. Good care of the dying patient. *JAMA.* 1996;275(6):474–478.

[49]Downing GM, Braithwaite DL, Wilde JM. Victoria BGY palliative care model—a new model for the 1990's. *J Palliat Care.* 1993;9(4):26–32.

[50]Doyle D. Domiciliary palliative care. In: Doyle D, Hanks G WC, MacDonald N, eds. *Oxford Textbook of Palliative Medicine.* New York: Oxford University Press; 1993:629–647.

[51]National Hospice Organization. Hospice awareness campaign "handle with care" needs your participation. *NHO Newsline.* 7(15):1.

[52]Kashiwagi T. Palliative care in Japan. *Palliat Med.* 1991;5:165–170.

[53]Kinzbrunner BM. Hospice: what to do when anti-cancer therapy is no longer appropriate, effective, or desired. *Sem Onc.* 1994:21(6):792–798.

[54]Mercadante S. Family doctor and palliative care team: 1988 versus 1990. *J Palliat Care.* 1991;7:38–39.

[55]Billings JA, Ferris FD, MacDonald N, von Gunten C. The role of palliative care in the home in medical education: report from a national consensus conference. *J Palliat Med.* 2001;4(3):361–371.

[56]Cassin CJ. Ethics of universal access to palliative care. Presented at Medicine at Life's End: Ethics and Humanities in Palliative Medicine. American Academy of Hospice and Palliative Medicine. March 14–15, 1997. Colorado Springs, Colo.

[57]Ham RJ. *Geriatrics I: AAFP Home Study Self-Assessment Monograph 89.* Kansas City, Mo.: American Academy of Family Practice; 1986. Cited by: Frederich ME. Physician home visits: a necessity, not a luxury. Presented at 9th Annual Assembly of the American Academy of Hospice and Palliative Medicine. Chicago. June 25–28, 1997.

[58]Irwin RS, Madison JM. Symptom research on chronic cough: a historical perspective. *Ann Intern Med.* 2001;134:809–814.

[59]Quill TE, Lo B, Block DW. Palliative options of last resort. *JAMA.* 1997;278:2009–2104.

[60]Quill TE, Lee BC, Nunn S. Palliative treatments of last resort: choosing the least harmful alternatives. *Ann Intern Med.* 2000;132:488–493.

[61]Prejean H. Keynote address to 1st national meeting on care of the dying in prisons and jails. Nov. 16,1998. www.soros.org/death/sisterhelen.htm. Accessed June 15, 2002.

[62]Craig EL, Craig RE. Prison hospice: an unlikely success. *Am J Hospice Palliat Care.* 1999;16(6):725–729.

[63]National Institute of Corrections. Hospice and palliative care in prisons. Special issues in corrections. Longmont, Colo.: NIC Information Center, 1998;2.

[64]Maull F. Issues in prison hospice: toward a model for the delivery of hospice care in a correctional setting. *Hospice J.* 1998;13(4):68–70.

[65]Seidlitz A. Doing "family" in a women's (prison) hospice. *NPHA News.* 1999; Spring 6:8–9.

[66]Brock DB, Foley DJ. Demography and epidemiology of dying in the US with emphasis on deaths of older persons. *Hospice J.* 1998;13:49–60.

[67]Miller SC, Mor V. The role of hospice care in the nursing home setting. *J Palliat Med.* 2002;5(2):271–277.

[68]Baer WM, Hanson LC. Families' perception of the added value of hospice in the nursing home. *J Am Geriatr Soc.* 2000;48:879–882.

[69]Miller SC, Gozalo P, Mor V. Hospice enrollment and hospitalization of dying nursing home residents. *Am J Med.* 2001;111:38–44.

[70]U.S. Department of Health and Human Services. Hospice patients in nursing homes. DHHS Publication No. OEI-05-95-00250, October, 1997.

[71]Government Accounting Office: Nursing home: additional steps needed to strengthen enforcement of federal quality standards. GAO.HEHS-99-46. March, 1999.

[72]Miller SC, Mor V, Wu N Gozalo P, Lapane K. Does receipt of hospice care in nursing homes improve the management of pain at the end-of-life? *J Am Geriatr Soc.* 2002:50(3)507–515.

[73]Angell M. Fixing Medicare. *N Engl J Med.* 1997;337(3):192–195.

[74]Vogelzang NJ, Chabner BA, Periman P, Ohrt DK, McCann BC, Burns JM, Bayer R. Reimbursement issues in clinical oncology. *Semin Oncol* 1988;15(suppl 6):S34–S43. Cited by: Joranson DE. Are health-care reimbursement policies a barrier to acute and cancer pain management? *J Pain Symptom Manage.* 1994;9(4):244–253.

[75]Von Gunten CF, Ferris FD, D'Antuono R, Emanuel LL. Recommendations to improve end-of-life care through regulatory change in U.S. health care financing. *J Palliat Med.* 2002;5(1):35–41.

[76]Lubitz JD, Riley GF. Trends in Medicare payments in the last year of life. *N Engl J Med.* 1993;328:1092–1096. Cited by: Emanuel E. Cost savings at the end of life: what do the data show? *JAMA.* 1996;275(24):1907–1914.

[77]Emanuel E. Cost savings at the end of life: what do the data show? *JAMA.* 1996;275(24):1907–1914.

[78]Iglehart JK. Health issues, the president, and the 105th congress. *N Engl J Med.* 1997; 336(9):671–675.

[79]1997 Annual Report to Congress. Washington, D.C.: Physician Payment Review Commission, 1997. Cited by: Angell M. Fixing Medicare. *N Engl J Med.* 1997;337(3):192–195.

[80]Levit KR, Lazenby HC, Braden BR, et al. National heath expenditures, 1995l Health Care Finance Rev. 1996; 18(1):175–214. Cited by: Angell M. Fixing Medicare. *N Engl J Med.* 1997;337(3):192–195.

[81]National Hospice Organization. *Hospice Fact Sheet.* Arlington, Va.: National Hospice Organization; July 1, 1996.

[82]*An Analysis of the Cost Savings of the Medicare Hospice Benefit.* Lewin-VHI, Inc. Arlington, Va.: National Hospice Organization. 1995.

[83]Cassel CK, Vladeck BC. ICD-9 code for palliative or terminal care. *N Engl J Med.* 1996;335(16):1232–1233.

[84]Navari RM, Stocking CB, Siegler M. Preferences of patients with advanced cancer for hospice care. *JAMA.* 2000;284:2449.

[85]Weeks JC, Cook F, O'Day SJ, et al. Relationships between cancer patients' predictions of prognosis and other treatment preferences. *JAMA.* 1998;279:1709–1714.

[86]Benefits Protection and Improvement Act, subtitle C, section 322, amending section 1814(a)(7) of the Social Security Act: as quoted in HCFA Program Memorandum to Intermediaries and Carriers, Transmittal AB-01-09, 1/24/01.

[87]Stuart B, Herbst L, Kinzbrunner B, Predor M, Connor S, Ryndes T. *Medical Guidelines for Determining Prognosis in Selected Non-Cancer Diseases,* 2nd ed. National Hospice Organization. 1901 North Moore Street, Suite 901, Arlington, Va., 1996.

[88]Stuart B. The NHO Medical Guidelines for Non-Cancer Disease and local medical review policy: hospice access for patients with diseases other than cancer. *Hospice J.* 1999;14:139–154.

[89]Schonwetter RS, Soendker S, Perron V, Martin B, Robinson BE, Thal AE. Review of Medicare's proposed hospital eligibility criteria for select noncancer patients. *Am J Hospice Palliat Care.* 1998;15:155–158.

[90]Zerzan J, Sterns S, Hanson L. Access to palliative care and hospice in nursing homes. *JAMA.* 2000;284: 2489–2494.

[91]Reimbursement for Hospice Care. *Medicare Hospice Manual.* §405. 02-90. Rev. 27.

[92]*1996 Green Book.* Center for Medicare and Medicaid Services, Baltimore, Md.

[93]Christakis NA, Escarce JJ. Survival of Medicare patients after enrollment in hospice programs. *N Engl J Med.* 1996;335(3):172–178.

[94]Medicare Hospice Conditions of Participation. Health Care Financing Administration. US Department of Health and Human Services. Memorandum, June 27, 1997.

[95]Q&A on Physician Care Plan Oversight. *NHO Newsline.* 1995;5(16):1. Arlington, Va.; National Hospice Organization.

[96]Roy DJ. Those days are long gone now. *J Palliat Care.* 1994;10(2):4–6.

[97]Heyland DK, Tranmer J, Feldman-Stewart DEB. End-of-life decision making in the seriously ill hospitalized patient: an organizing framework and results of a preliminary study. *J Palliat Care.* 2000;16:531–539.

[98]National Hospice Organization. *Discontinuation of Hospice Care; Ethical Issues.* Arlington, Va.: National Hospice Organization; 1993.

[99]Brenner PR. Issues of access in a diverse society. *Hospice J.* 1997;12(2):9–16.

[100]Gordon AK. Hospice and minorities: a national study of organizational access and practice. *Hospice J.* 1996;11(1):49–70.

[101]Craig EL, Craig RE. Prison hospice: an unlikely success. *Am J Hosp Palliat Care.* 1999;16:725–729.

[102]Bruera E. Research in symptoms other than pain. In: Doyle D, Hanks GWC, MacDonald N, eds. *Oxford Textbook of Palliative Medicine.* New York: Oxford University Press; 1993:87–92.

[103]Liaison Committee on Medical Education 1992–1993 Annual Medical School Questionnaire, Part II. Reported by: Council on Scientific Affairs, American Medical Association. Good care of the dying patient. *JAMA.* 1996;275(6):474–478.

[104]Martini CJM, Grenholm G. Institutional responsibility in graduate medical education and highlights of historical data. *JAMA.* 1993;270:1053–1060. Cited by: Council on Scientific Affairs, American Medical Association. Good care of the dying patient. *JAMA.* 1996;275(6):474–478.

[105]Scott JF, MacDonald N. Education in palliative medicine. In: *Oxford Textbook of Palliative Medicine*, eds. Doyle D, Hanks GWC, MacDonald N. New York: Oxford University Press; 1993:761–781.

[106]Knight, CF, Knight PF, Gellula M, Holman GH. Training our future physicians: a hospice rotation for medical students. *Am J Hospice and Palliat Care.* 1992;9(1):23–28.

[107]*Caring for the Dying: Identification and Promotion of Physician Competency.* Philadelphia, Pa: American Board of Internal Medicine. 1996.

[108]Billings JA, Block S. Palliative care in undergraduate medical education: status report and future directions. *JAMA.* 1997;278(9):733–738.

[109]Matinez JM, Neely KJ, Preodor ME, Twaddle M, von Gunten C. *Teaching Hospice/Palliative Care.* Presented at the 9th Annual Assembly of the American Academy of Hospice and Palliative Medicine. Chicago. June 25–28, 1997.

[110]Weissman DE, Block SD, Blank L, Cain J, Cassem N, Danoff D, Foley K, Meier D, Schyve P, Theige D, Wheeler HB. Recommendations for incorporating palliative care education into the acute care hospital setting. *Acad Med.* 1999;74:871–877.

[111]Bruera E. Ethical issues in palliative care. *J Palliat Care.* 1994;10(3):7–9.

[112]Max MB, Portenoy RK. Pain research: designing clinical trials in palliative care. In: Doyle D, Hanks GWC, MacDonald N, eds. *Oxford Textbook of Palliative Medicine.* New York: Oxford University Press; 1993:77–86.

[113]Cleeland CS, Mendoza TR, Wang XS, Chou C, Harle MT, Morrissey M, Engstrom MC. Assessing symptom distress in cancer patients: the M.D. Anderson Symptom Inventory. *Cancer.* 2000;89:1634–1646.

[114]Kristjanson LJ. Research in palliative care populations: ethical issues. *J Palliat Care.* 1994;10(3):10–15.

[115]Alexander DA. Psychological/social research. In: Doyle D, Hanks GWC, MacDonald N, eds. *Oxford Textbook of Palliative Medicine.* New York: Oxford University Press; 1993:92–96.

[116]Corless I. The hospice movement in North America. In: Corr C, Corr D, eds. *Hospice Care: Principles and Practice.* New York: Springer Publishing Co.: 1983. Cited by: Campbell L. History of the hospice movement. *Cancer Nurs.* 1986;9(6):333–338.

[117]Beresford L. The future of hospice in a reformed American health care system: what are the real questions? *Hospice J.* 1997;12(2):85–91.

[118]Council on Scientific Affairs, American Medical Association. Good care of the dying patient. *JAMA.* 1996;275(6):474–478.

[119]von Gunten CF, Sloan P, Portenoy R, Schonwetter R. Physician board certification in hospice and palliative medicine. *J Palliat Med.* 2000;3:441–447.

[120]Kroenke K. Studying symptoms: sampling and measurement issues. *Ann Intern Med.* 2001;134:844–853.

[121]Mahoney JJ. Hospice and managed care. *Hospice J.* 1997;12(2):81–84.

[122]Anders G. HMOs pile-up billions in cash, try to decide what to do with it. *Wall Street Journal.* December 21, 1994:A1. Cited by: Showstack J, Lurie N, Leatherman S, Fisher E, Inui T. Health of the public: the private-sector challenge. *JAMA.* 1996;276(13):1071–1074.

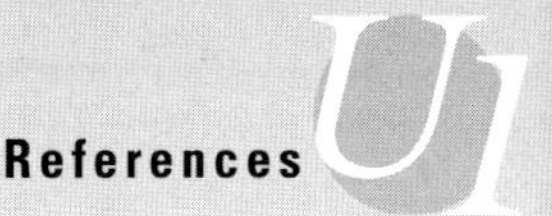

[123]Group Health Association of America. *Patterns in HMO Enrollment.* Washington, D.C.: Groups Health Association of America; June 1995. Cited by: Ware JE, Bayliss MS, Rogers WH, Kosinski M, Tarlov AR. Differences in 4-year health outcomes for elderly and poor, chronically ill patients treated in HMO and fee-for-services systems. *JAMA.* 1996;276(13):1039–1047.

[124]Morgan RO, Virnig BA, DeVito CA, Persily NA. The Medicare-HMO revolving door—the healthy go in and the sick go out. *N Engl J Med.* 1997;337(3):169–175.

[125]Ware JE, Bayliss MS, Rogers WH, Kosinski M, Tarlov AR. Differences in 4-year health outcomes for elderly and poor, chronically ill patients treated in HMO and fee-for-services systems. *JAMA.* 1996;276(13):1039–1047.

[126]Annas GJ. Patients' rights in managed care—exit, voice, and choice. *N Engl J Med.* 1997;337(3):210–215.

[127]Inglehart JK. Medicaid and managed care. *N Engl J Med.* 1995;332:1727–1731. Cited by: Showstack J, Lurie N, Leatherman S, Fisher E, Inui T. Health of the public: the private-sector challenge. *JAMA.* 1996;276(13):1071–1074.

[128]Addington-Hall J, Fakhoury W, McCarthy M. Specialist palliative care in nonmalignant disease. *Palliat Med.* 1998;12:417–427.

[129]Jones AB, Moga DI, Davie KA. Transforming end-of-life care for the 21st century: the hospice vision. *J Palliat Med.* 1999;2:9–14.

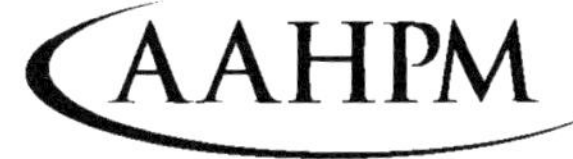

**American Academy of Hospice and Palliative Medicine**

*UNIPAC One: The Hospice/Palliative Medicine Approach to End-of-Life Care*

Physicians are eligible to receive 6 credit hours in Category 1 of the AMA/PRA by completing and returning this posttest answer sheet to the AAHPM. The Academy will keep a record of AMA/PRA Category 1 credit hours and the record will be provided on request; however, physicians are responsible for reporting their own Category 1 CME credits when applying for the AMA/PRA or for other certificates or credentials.

Name ____________________

Street ____________________

City/State/Zip Code ____________________

Telephone ____________________

Social Security Number ____________________

*Please mail this answer sheet and a check for $45.00 made out to the American Academy of Hospice and Palliative Medicine to:*

***Physician Training Programs***
***American Academy of Hospice and Palliative Medicine***
***4700 W. Lake Avenue***
***Glenview, Illinois 60023-1485***

Please circle the one correct answer for each question

| | | | | | | | | |
|---|---|---|---|---|---|---|---|---|
| 1. | A | B | C | D | 13. | A | B | C | D |
| 2. | A | B | C | D | 14. | A | B | C | D |
| 3. | A | B | C | D | 15. | A | B | C | D |
| 4. | A | B | C | D | 16. | A | B | C | D |
| 5. | A | B | C | D | 17. | A | B | C | D |
| 6. | A | B | C | D | 18. | A | B | C | D |
| 7. | A | B | C | D | 19. | A | B | C | D |
| 8. | A | B | C | D | 20. | A | B | C | D |
| 9. | A | B | C | D | 21. | A | B | C | D |
| 10. | A | B | C | D | 22. | A | B | C | D |
| 11. | A | B | C | D | 23. | A | B | C | D |
| 12. | A | B | C | D | 24. | A | B | C | D |